What's New in this Edition?

Stretching is one of the most popular fitness books of all time. It has sold 3¾ million copies worldwide and is in 24 languages.

Stretching Pocket Book – 40th Anniversary Edition has been updated with:

- New stretching routines for smartphone users
- Suggestions for dealing with the conditions known as "tech neck" and "text neck"
- Tips on improving posture

* * * *

Stretching is a simple, gentle activity that can be done by anyone, anywhere, at any time.

This second edition of *Pocket Book – 40th Anniversary Edition* contains:

- 150 stretches with simple instructions for each stretch
- One- or two-page graphic stretching ~~routines~~
- 17 routines for ever~~
- 10 routines for com~~
- 37 routines for diffe~~
- Graphic index of all 15~~ ~~cal profes-
sions, and body work~~ ~~for patients
- Body tools
- Caring for your back
- PNF stretching

You can make photocopies of different routines for easy reference. Just the one page will give you a series of stretches tailored to your individual needs. Keep in a desk drawer or put on the wall or floor when stretching.

If you stretch in the right way (no bouncing, no pain), you'll feel better. It's that simple.

–Bob and Jean Anderson

Bob
Jean

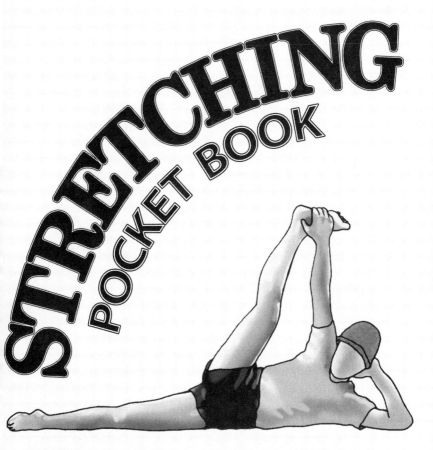

STRETCHING
POCKET BOOK

40th Anniversary Edition

BOB ANDERSON
Illustrated by JEAN ANDERSON

Shelter Publications, Inc.
Bolinas, California
www.shelterpub.com

Distributed in the United States by Publishers Group West and in Canada by Publishers Group Canada

Library of Congress Control Number: 2021933386

1 — 21
(Lowest digits indicate number and year of latest printing.)

Printed in the United States of America

Shelter Publications, Inc.
P.O. Box 279
Bolinas, California 94924
415-868-0280
Email: shelter@shelterpub.com

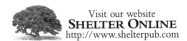

Visit our website
SHELTER ONLINE
http://www.shelterpub.com

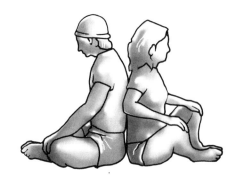

Contents

Stretching in the Age of Computers and Smartphones..... 138

Stretching Routines: Sports 154

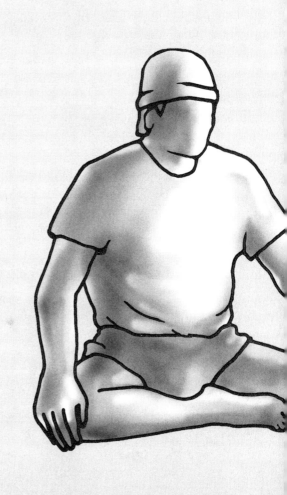

GETTING STARTED

This first section is an introduction to stretching. It is very important to read pages 12–13, "How to Stretch," so you will understand how to do the stretches in the rest of the book. Then, if you are new to stretching, the section "Getting Started," on pages 15–21, will take you through a series of simple stretches.

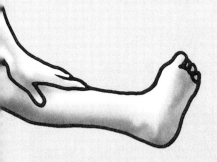

INTRODUCTION

Today millions of people have discovered the benefits of movement. Everywhere you look they are out: running, cycling, skating, playing tennis, or swimming. What do they hope to accomplish? Why this relatively sudden interest in physical fitness?

Many recent studies have shown that active people lead fuller lives. They have more stamina, resist illness, and stay trim. They have more self-confidence, are less depressed, and often, even late in life, are still working energetically on new projects.

Medical research has shown that a great deal of ill health is directly related to lack of physical activity. We now realize that the only way to prevent the diseases of inactivity is to remain active — not for a month, or a year, but for a lifetime.

* * * *

Our ancestors did not have the problems that go with a sedentary life; they had to work hard to survive. They stayed strong and healthy through continuous, vigorous outdoor work: chopping, digging, tilling, planting, hunting, etc. But with the advent of the Industrial Revolution, machines began to do the work once done by hand. As people became less active, they began to lose strength and flexibility.

Machines have obviously made life easier, but they have also created serious problems. Instead of walking, we drive; rather than climb stairs, we use elevators. Computers have made us even more sedentary. Without daily physical exertion, our bodies become storehouses of unreleased tensions. With no natural outlets for our tensions, our muscles become weak and tight, and we lose touch with our physical nature.

Health is something we can control. We are no longer content to sit and stagnate. Now we are moving, rediscovering the joys of an active, healthy life. What's more, we can resume a more healthy and rewarding existence at any age.

* * * *

The body's capacity for recovery is phenomenal. For example, a surgeon makes an incision, removes or corrects the problem, then sews you back up. At this point, the body takes over and heals itself. All of us have this seemingly miraculous capacity for regaining health, whether it's from something as drastic as surgery, or from poor physical condition caused by lack of activity and bad diet.

What does stretching have to do with all this? It is the important link between the sedentary life and the active life. It keeps the muscles supple, prepares you for movement, and helps you make the daily transition from inactivity to vigorous activity without undue strain. It is especially important if you run, cycle, play tennis, or engage in sports, because activities like these promote tightness and inflexibility.

Stretching is easy, but when it is done incorrectly, it can actually do more harm than good. For this reason it is essential to understand the right techniques.

* * * *

Stretching feels good when done correctly. You do not have to push limits or attempt to go further each day. It should not be a personal contest to see how far you can stretch. Stretching should be tailored to your particular muscular structure, flexibility, and varying tension levels. The key is regularity and relaxation. The object is to reduce muscular tension, thereby promoting freer movement — not to concentrate on attaining extreme flexibility, which often leads to overstretching and injury.

We can learn a lot by observing animals. Watch a cat. It instinctively knows how to stretch. It does so spontaneously, never overstretching, continually and naturally tuning up muscles it will have to use.

* * * *

Stretching is not stressful. It is peaceful, relaxing, and noncompetitive. The subtle, invigorating feelings of stretching allow you to get in touch with your muscles. It is completely adjustable to the individual. You do not have to conform to any unyielding discipline; stretching gives you the freedom to be yourself and enjoy being yourself.

Anyone can be fit, with the right approach. You don't need to be a great athlete. But you do need to take it slowly, especially in the beginning. Give your body and mind time to adjust to the stresses of physical activity. Start easily and be regular. There is no way to get into shape in a day.

When you are stretching regularly and exercising frequently, you will learn to enjoy movement. Remember that each one of us is a unique physical and mental being with our own comfortable and enjoyable rhythms. We are all different in strength, endurance, flexibility, and temperament. If you learn about your body and its needs, you will be able to develop your own personal potential and gradually build a foundation of fitness that will last a lifetime.

Who Should Stretch

Everyone can learn to stretch, regardless of age or flexibility. You do not need to be in top physical condition or have specific athletic skills. Whether you sit at a desk all day, dig ditches, do housework, stand at an assembly line, drive a truck, or exercise regularly, the same techniques of stretching apply. The methods are gentle and easy, conforming to individual differences in muscle tension and flexibility. So, if you are healthy, without any specific physical problems, you can learn how to stretch safely and enjoyably.

> **Note:** If you have had any recent physical problems or surgery, particularly of the joints and muscles, or if you have been inactive or sedentary for some time, please consult your health care professional before you start a stretching or exercise program.

When to Stretch

Stretching can be done any time you feel like it: at work, in a car, waiting for a bus, walking down the road, under a nice shady tree after a hike, or at the beach. Stretch before and after physical activity, but also stretch at various times of the day when you can. Here are some examples:

- In the morning before the start of the day
- At work to release nervous tension
- After sitting or standing for a long time
- When you feel stiff
- At odd times during the day, as for instance, when watching TV, listening to music, reading, or sitting and talking

Why Stretch

Stretching, because it relaxes your mind and tunes up your body, should be part of your daily life. You will find that regular stretching will do the following things:

- Reduce muscle tension and make the body feel more relaxed
- Help coordination by allowing for freer and easier movement
- Increase range of motion
- Help prevent injuries such as muscle strains. (A strong, flexible, pre-stretched muscle resists stress better than a strong, stiff, unstretched muscle.)
- Make strenuous activities like running, skiing, tennis, swimming, and cycling easier because it prepares you for activity; it's a way of signaling the muscles that they are about to be used.
- Help maintain your current level of flexibility, so as time passes you do not become stiffer and stiffer
- Develop body awareness; as you stretch various parts of the body, you focus on them and get in touch with them; you get to know yourself.
- Help loosen the mind's control of the body so that the body moves for "its own sake" rather than for competition or ego
- Feel good

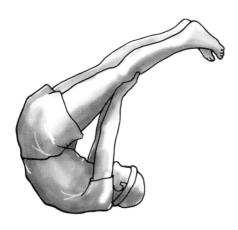

How to Stretch

Stretching is easy to learn. But there is a right way and a wrong way to stretch. The right way is a relaxed, sustained stretch with your attention focused on the muscles being stretched. The wrong way (unfortunately practiced by many people) is to bounce up and down or to stretch to the point of pain: these methods can actually do more harm than good.

If you stretch correctly and regularly, you will find that every movement you make becomes easier. It will take time to loosen up tight muscles or muscle groups, but time is quickly forgotten when you start to feel good.

The Easy Stretch

When you begin a stretch, spend 5–15 seconds in the *easy stretch*. No bouncing! Go to the point where you feel a *mild tension,* and relax as you hold the stretch. The feeling of tension should subside as you hold the position. If it does not, ease off slightly and find a degree of tension that is comfortable. You should be able to say, "I feel the stretch, but it is not painful." The easy stretch reduces muscular tightness and tension and readies the tissues for the developmental stretch.

The Developmental Stretch

After the easy stretch, move slowly into the *developmental stretch.* Again, no bouncing. Move a fraction of an inch further until you again feel a mild tension and hold for 5–15 seconds. Be in control. Again, the tension should diminish; if not, ease off slightly. Remember: If the stretch tension increases as the stretch is held and/or it becomes painful, you are stretching too far! The developmental stretch fine-tunes the muscles and increases flexibility.

Breathing

Your breathing should be slow, rhythmical, and under control. If you are bending forward to do a stretch, exhale as you bend forward and then breathe slowly as you hold the stretch. Do not hold your breath while stretching. If a stretch position inhibits your natural breathing pattern, then you are obviously not relaxed. Just ease up on the stretch so you can breathe naturally.

Counting

At first, silently count the seconds for each stretch; this will insure that you hold the proper tension for a long enough time. After a while, you will be stretching by the way it feels, without the distraction of counting.

The Stretch Reflex

Your muscles are protected by a mechanism called the *stretch reflex*. Any time you stretch the muscle fibers too far (either by bouncing or over-stretching), a nerve reflex responds by sending a signal to the muscles to contract; this keeps the muscles from being injured. Thus, stretching too far tightens the very muscles you are trying to stretch! (You get a similar involuntary muscle reaction when you accidentally touch something hot; before you can think about it, your body jerks away from the heat.)

Pushing a stretch too far or bouncing up and down strains the muscles and activates the stretch reflex. This causes pain, as well as physical damage due to the microscopic tearing of muscle fibers. This in turn leads to the formation of scar tissue in the muscles, with a gradual loss of elasticity. The muscles become stiff and sore. It's hard to get enthused about daily stretching and exercise when you're pushing it to the point of pain!

No Gain *with* Pain

Many of us were conditioned in high school to the idea of "no gain without pain." We learned to associate pain with physical improvement, and were taught that ". . . the more it hurts, the more you get out of it." Don't be fooled. Stretching, when done correctly, is not painful. Learn to pay attention to your body, for pain is an indication that something is *wrong*.

The easy and developmental stretches, as described on the previous page, do not overactivate the stretch reflex and do not cause pain.

This Diagram Will Give You an Idea of a "Good Stretch"

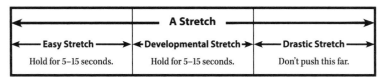

	A Stretch	
← Easy Stretch →	← Developmental Stretch →	← Drastic Stretch →
Hold for 5–15 seconds.	Hold for 5–15 seconds.	Don't push this far.

The straight-line diagram represents the stretch that is possible with your muscles and their connective tissue. You will find that your flexibility will naturally increase when you stretch, first in the easy, then in the developmental phase. By stretching regularly and staying relaxed, you will be able to go beyond your present limits and come closer to your personal potential.

Warming Up and Cooling Down

Warming Up

There has been some controversy in recent years about stretching before you warm up. If you are going to stretch, will you get injured if you stretch without specifically warming up first? No — if you stretch comfortably and not strenuously. However, I suggest that you do several minutes of general movement (walking and swinging arms, etc.) to warm the muscles and related soft tissue before you stretch. This will get the blood moving. You still have to stretch correctly whether you are warmed up or not.

Some runners have reported they are more likely to get injured if they don't warm up before stretching. It is possible to get hurt stretching if:
• you are in too much of a hurry (not relaxed)
• you push too far, too soon (overstretching a cold muscle)
• you are not paying attention to the feeling of the stretch

You will not get hurt stretching if you stretch correctly *(see pp. 12–13).* You will sense how far to stretch if you are paying attention to how the stretch feels; tune in to your body.

Here's my advice if you are engaging in an activity such as running or cycling or whatever: Warm up by doing the activity you are about to do, but at a lower intensity. For example, if you are about to run — walk or jog for 2–5 minutes or until you break a light sweat. (Walking and jogging provide a good, basic warm-up for many activities. This will increase muscle and blood temperature and raise total body temperature to provide an effective warm-up.) Then stretch. After you have stretched, continue to warm up for another 5 minutes or so to complete a full warm-up.

Cooling Down

Conversely, you should cool down after exercise by doing a scaled-down version of the main workout. Get your heart rate back down towards a resting rate. Then stretch to prevent muscle soreness and stiffness.

Getting Started

Here we will walk you through nine stretches that will help you to understand the phrase "Go with the *feel* of the stretch." Once you understand this technique, it will be easy to learn and use the stretches in this book.

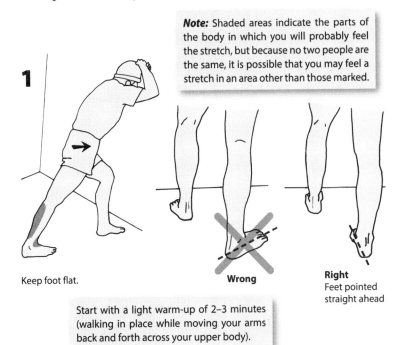

Note: Shaded areas indicate the parts of the body in which you will probably feel the stretch, but because no two people are the same, it is possible that you may feel a stretch in an area other than those marked.

Keep foot flat.

Wrong

Right
Feet pointed straight ahead

Start with a light warm-up of 2–3 minutes (walking in place while moving your arms back and forth across your upper body).

First we'll do a calf stretch.

• Stand a little way from wall and lean on it with forearms, head resting on hands.
• Place left foot in front of you, leg bent, right leg straight behind you.
• Slowly move hips forward until you feel stretch in calf of right leg.
• Keep right heel flat and toes pointed straight ahead.
• Hold easy stretch 5–10 seconds.
• Do not bounce.
• Repeat on other side.

Now stretch the other calf. Does one leg feel different from the other? Is one leg more flexible than the other?

Sitting Groin Stretch:

- Sit on floor, soles of feet together; hold onto toes and feet.
- Gently pull forward, bending from hips.

- Hold 5–15 seconds. Do not bounce.
- Keep elbows on outside of lower legs.
- Breathe slowly and deeply.

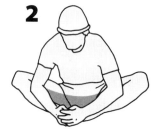

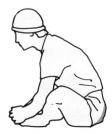

Exhale as you go into the stretch. Breathe slowly and rhythmically as you hold it. Relax your jaw and shoulders.

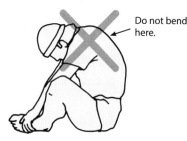

Do not bend here.

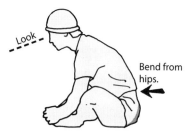

Look

Bend from hips.

Do not bend forward from your head and shoulders. This rounds the shoulders and puts pressure on lower back.

Concentrate on making the initial move forward from your hips. Keep your lower back flat. Look out in front of you.

After you feel the tension diminish slightly, increase the stretch by gently pulling yourself a little further into the stretch feeling. Now it should feel a bit more intense *but not painful.* Hold for about 15 seconds. The feeling of tension should decrease slightly the longer the stretch is held. Slowly come out of the stretch. Please, no jerky, quick, bouncing movements!

> Stretch by the *feel* of the stretch, not by how *far* you can stretch.

3

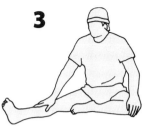

- Straighten right leg as you keep left leg bent.
- Sole of the left foot should be facing inside of right upper leg.
- Do not "lock" straight leg.

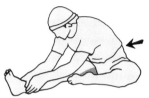

- To stretch hamstrings and left side of lower back, bend forward from hips until you feel slight stretch.
- Hold 5–15 seconds.
- Touch quadriceps of right thigh to make sure these muscles are relaxed. They should be soft, not tight.

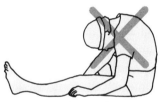

Don't make the initial movement with your head and shoulders. Don't try to touch your forehead to your knee. This will only round your shoulders.

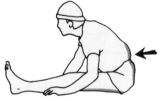

Do initiate the stretch from the hips. Keep your chin in a neutral position. Keep your shoulders and arms relaxed.

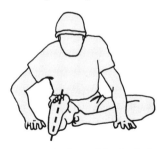

Be sure the foot of the leg being stretched is upright, with the ankle and toes relaxed. This will keep you aligned through the ankle, knee, and hip.

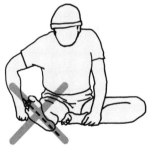

Do not let your leg turn to the outside because this causes misalignment of the leg and hip.

If you are not very flexible, use a towel around the bottom of your foot to do this stretch.

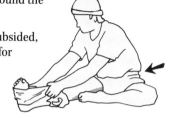

After the feeling of the easy stretch has subsided, slowly go into the developmental stretch for 5–15 seconds. You may only have to bend forward a fraction of an inch. Do not worry about how far you can go. Remember, we are all different.

Slowly come out of the stretch. Do the same stretch on the other side. Keep the front of your thigh relaxed and your foot upright, with ankle and toes relaxed. Do an easy stretch for 15 seconds, and then slowly find the developmental phase of the stretch and hold for 5–15 seconds.

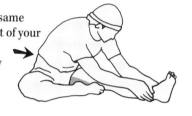

It takes time and sensitivity to stretch properly.

Develop your ability to stretch by how you feel and not by how far you can stretch.

4

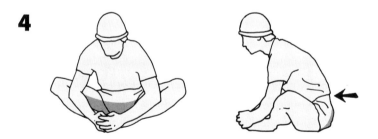

Repeat the sitting groin stretch. How does this feel as compared to the first time you did it? Any change at all?

A number of things are more important than concentrating solely on increasing flexibility:

1. Relaxation of tense areas such as feet, hands, wrists, shoulders, and jaw when stretching

2. Learning how to find and control the right amount of tension in each stretch

3. Awareness of lower back, head and shoulders, and leg alignment during the stretch

4. Adjusting to daily changes, for every day the body feels slightly different

5

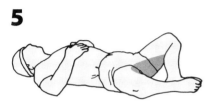

Lying Groin Stretch:
- Lie on floor and relax.
- Bend knees, soles of feet together.
- Lower knees out to sides.
- Let gravity do the stretching.
- Hold 10–30 seconds.

Let go of any tension. The stretch feeling here will be subtle.

6

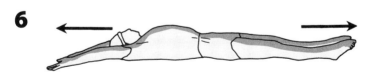

Elongation Stretch:
- Lie on floor, extend arms overhead, keep legs straight.
- Reach arms and legs in opposite directions.
- Stretch 5 seconds; relax.
- Gently pull in your abdominal muscles to make the middle of your body thin.
- A great stretch to do first thing in the morning while still in bed.

7

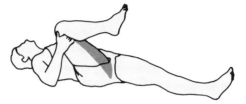

- Lie on floor, legs straight or with one leg bent *(optional)*.
- Gently pull right knee to chest.
- Hold 10–30 seconds; relax.
- Repeat for other leg.

Gradually get to know yourself.

8

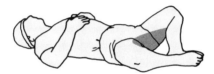

Repeat the lying groin stretch and relax for 30 seconds. Let go of any tension in your feet, hands, and shoulders. You may want to do this stretch with your eyes closed.

How to Sit Up from a Lying Position

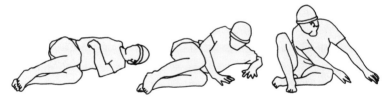

Bend both knees and roll over onto one side. While resting on your side, use your hands to push yourself up into a sitting position. By using your hands and arms this way, you take the pressure or stress off the back.

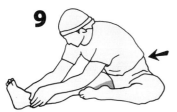

9 Now repeat the stretches for your hamstrings. Have you changed at all? Do you feel more limber and less tense than before stretching?

SUMMARY

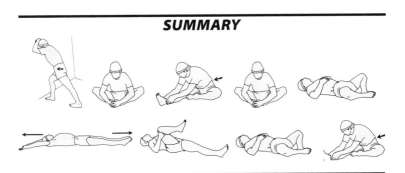

These are just a few stretches to get you started. I want you to understand that stretching is not a contest in flexibility. Your flexibility will naturally improve with proper stretching. Stretch with feelings you can enjoy.

After a while the amount of time (20–30 seconds) you hold stretches will vary. Sometimes you may want to hold a stretch longer because you are extra tight that day, or you are just enjoying the stretch. Or you may not want to hold a stretch as long when your body already feels fairly limber; this would generally be when you hold a stretch for 5–15 seconds. *Remember that no two days are the same* so you must gauge your stretching by how you feel at the moment.

THE STRETCHES

In the following section (pp. 26–103) are all the stretches in the book, with instructions for each position. They are grouped according to body parts and presented as a series, but any of them may be done separately without doing the entire routine.

Note: You need not stretch as far as the drawings indicate. Stretch by how you feel without trying to imitate the figure in the drawings. Adjust each stretch to your own personal flexibility, which will vary daily.

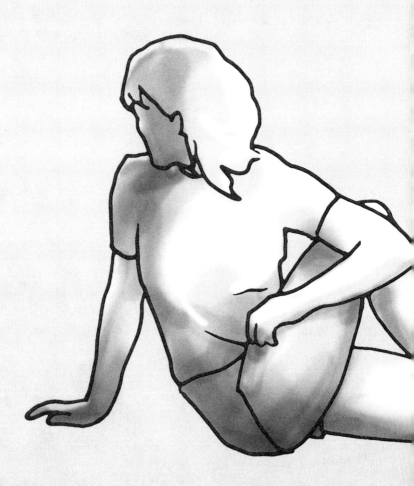

Learn stretches for the various parts of the body, at first concentrating on the areas of greatest tension or tightness. On the next two pages is a guide to various muscles and body parts, with reference to the page where each may be found in the book.

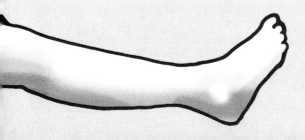

Stretching Guide

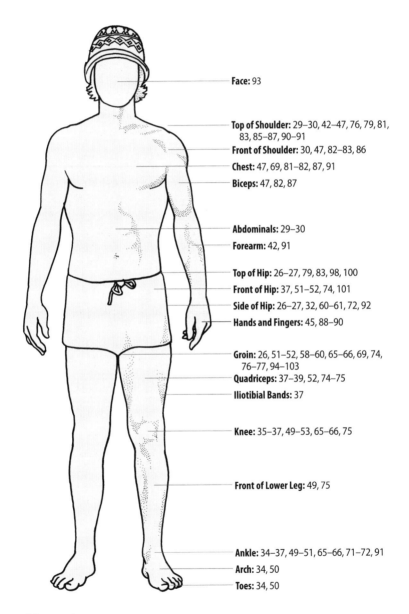

Face: 93

Top of Shoulder: 29–30, 42–47, 76, 79, 81, 83, 85–87, 90–91
Front of Shoulder: 30, 47, 82–83, 86
Chest: 47, 69, 81–82, 87, 91
Biceps: 47, 82, 87

Abdominals: 29–30
Forearm: 42, 91

Top of Hip: 26–27, 79, 83, 98, 100
Front of Hip: 37, 51–52, 74, 101
Side of Hip: 26–27, 32, 60–61, 72, 92
Hands and Fingers: 45, 88–90

Groin: 26, 51–52, 58–60, 65–66, 69, 74, 76–77, 94–103
Quadriceps: 37–39, 52, 74–75
Iliotibial Bands: 37

Knee: 35–37, 49–53, 65–66, 75

Front of Lower Leg: 49, 75

Ankle: 34–37, 49–51, 65–66, 71–72, 91
Arch: 34, 50
Toes: 34, 50

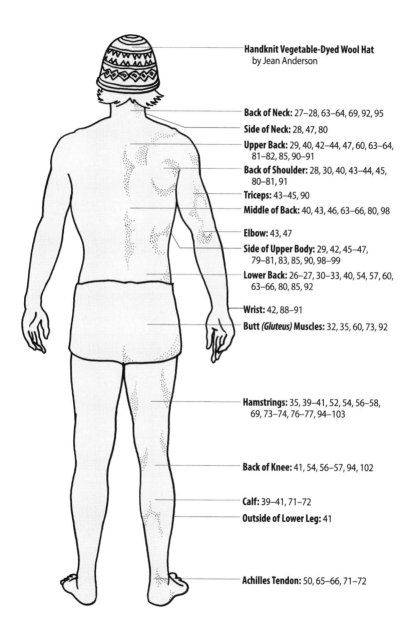

Handknit Vegetable-Dyed Wool Hat
by Jean Anderson

Back of Neck: 27–28, 63–64, 69, 92, 95

Side of Neck: 28, 47, 80

Upper Back: 29, 40, 42–44, 47, 60, 63–64, 81–82, 85, 90–91

Back of Shoulder: 28, 30, 40, 43–44, 45, 80–81, 91

Triceps: 43–45, 90

Middle of Back: 40, 43, 46, 63–66, 80, 98

Elbow: 43, 47

Side of Upper Body: 29, 42, 45–47, 79–81, 83, 85, 90, 98–99

Lower Back: 26–27, 30–33, 40, 54, 57, 60, 63–66, 80, 85, 92

Wrist: 42, 88–91

Butt (*Gluteus*) Muscles: 32, 35, 60, 73, 92

Hamstrings: 35, 39–41, 52, 54, 56–58, 69, 73–74, 76–77, 94–103

Back of Knee: 41, 54, 56–57, 94, 102

Calf: 39–41, 71–72

Outside of Lower Leg: 41

Achilles Tendon: 50, 65–66, 71–72

Relaxing Stretches for Your Back

This is a series of very easy stretches that you can do lying on your back. This series is beneficial because each position stretches a body area that is generally hard to relax. You can use this routine for mild stretching and relaxation.

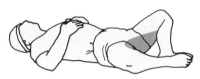

- Lie on floor and relax.
- Bend knees, soles of feet together.
- Lower knees out to sides.
- Let gravity do the stretching.
- Hold 10–30 seconds.

Variation:

- From this lying groin stretch, gently rock your legs as one unit *(see dotted lines)* back and forth about 10–12 times.
- These are real easy movements of no more than 1″ in either direction.
- Initiate movements from top of your hips.
- Will gently limber up your groin and hips.

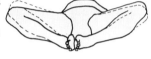

A Stretch for the Lower Back, Side, and Top of Hip

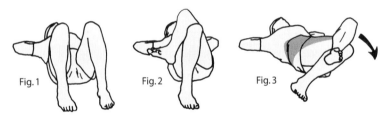

Fig. 1   Fig. 2   Fig. 3

- Lie on floor, fingers interlaced behind head.
- Bend knees, cross left leg over right knee.
- Use left leg to pull right leg toward floor until you feel mild stretch along side of hip and lower back.
- Keep upper back, shoulders, and elbows flat on floor.
- Stretch knee toward floor.
- Hold 10–20 seconds.
- Repeat on other side.

- Do not hold your breath.
- Breathe rhythmically.
- Relax.

If you have sciatic* problems of the lower back, this stretch can help. But *be careful*. Hold only stretch tensions that feel good. Never stretch to the point of pain.

PNF Technique: *Contract — Relax — Stretch. (See pp. 235–239.)*

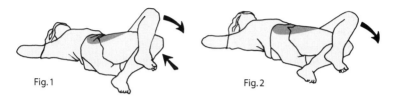

Fig. 1   Fig. 2

- Lie on floor, bend knees, keep feet flat.
- Interlace fingers behind head at ear level.
- Use arms to gently pull head forward, feel slight stretch.
- Hold 4–5 seconds, relax.
- Repeat 3 times.

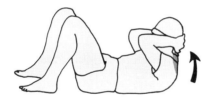

To reduce tension in the neck:

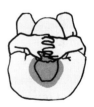

- While still lying on the floor, you can stretch upper spine and neck.
- Interlace fingers behind head at about ear level.
- Slowly pull head forward until you feel a slight stretch in back of neck.
- Hold 3–5 seconds, then slowly return to original starting position.
- Do 3–4 times to loosen up upper spine and neck gradually.
- Keep jaw relaxed (back teeth slightly separated) and keep breathing.

---

*The sciatic nerve is the longest and largest nerve of the body. It originates in the lumbar portion of the spine (lower back) and travels down the entire length of both legs and out to the great toe.

PNF Technique: *Contract — Relax — Stretch.*

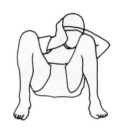

- From a bent-knee position, interlace fingers behind head (not neck).
- Before stretching back of neck, gently lift head upward and forward off floor.
- Move back of head downward toward floor as you resist movement with hands and arms.
- Hold this isometric contraction for 3–4 seconds.
- Relax 1–2 seconds, then gently pull head forward (as in previous stretch), with chin going toward navel until you feel a mild, comfortable stretch.
- Hold 3–5 seconds.
- Do 2–3 times.

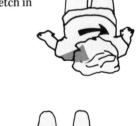

- Gently pull head and chin toward left knee.
- Hold for 3–5 seconds.
- Relax and lower head back down to floor.
- Pull head gently toward right knee.
- Repeat 2–3 times.

- With back of head on floor, turn chin toward shoulder (keep head resting on floor).
- Turn chin only as far as needed to get easy stretch in side of neck.
- Hold 3–5 seconds, then stretch to other side.
- Repeat 2–3 times.
- Keep jaw relaxed and don't hold breath.

Shoulder Blade Pinch:

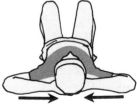

- Lie on floor, bend knees, feet flat.
- Interlace fingers behind head at ear level.
- Bring shoulder blades toward each other until tension is felt.
- Hold 4–5 seconds; relax and repeat.

Think of creating tension in neck and shoulders, relaxing same area, then stretching back of neck to help keep muscles of neck free to move without tightness. Repeat 3–4 times.

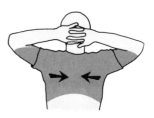

Lower Back Flattener:

- To relieve tension in lower back, tighten butt *(gluteus)* muscles and, at same time, tighten abdominal muscles to flatten lower back.
- Hold tension 5–8 seconds; relax.
- Repeat 2–3 times.
- Concentrate on maintaining constant muscle contraction.

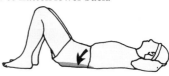

This pelvic tilting exercise will strengthen butt *(gluteus)* and abdominal muscles so you are able to sit and stand with good posture.

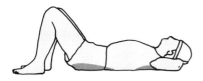
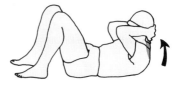

Shoulder Blade Pinch and Gluteus Tightener:

- Lie on floor, bend knees, keep feet flat.
- Interlace fingers behind head at ear level.
- Use arms to gently pull head forward; feel slight stretch.

- Tighten butt muscles.
- Hold 4–5 seconds; relax.
- Repeat 3 times.

- Lie on floor, bend knees.
- Extend one arm above head (palm up), other arm at side (palm down).
- Reach arms in opposite directions.
- Hold 5 seconds; both sides twice.
- Keep lower back relaxed, flat on floor.
- Keep jaw relaxed.

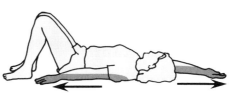

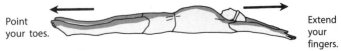

Point your toes.   Extend your fingers.

Elongation Stretches:

- Lie on floor, extend arms overhead, keep legs straight.
- Reach arms and legs in opposite directions.
- Stretch 5 seconds; relax.

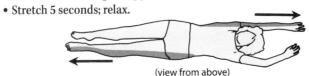

(view from above)

- Lie on floor, legs straight.
- Extend right arm above head (palms up), left arm by side, palm down.
- Stretch diagonally.

- Point toes of left foot as you extend right arm.
- Stretch as far as is comfortable.
- Hold 5 seconds, then relax.
- Reverse and stretch left arm and point toes of right foot.

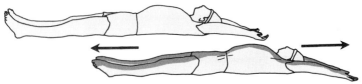

- Stretch both arms and both legs again, at same time.
- Hold 5 seconds; relax.
- Good stretch for muscles of rib cage, abdominals, spine, shoulders, arms, ankles, and feet.

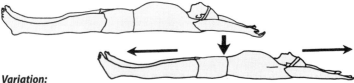

Variation:

- Pull in with abdominal muscles while stretching.
- Will make you feel slim, and is great exercise for internal organs.
- Doing elongation stretches 3 times reduces tension and tightness and relaxes spine and entire body.
- Helps to reduce overall body tension quickly.
- Do just before sleeping.

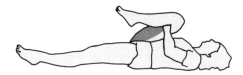

- Lie on floor, legs straight or with one leg bent *(optional)*.
- Gently pull with both hands behind right knee to chest.
- Keep lower back flat.
- Hold 10–30 seconds; relax.
- Repeat other leg.

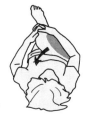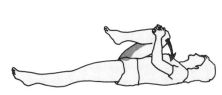

Variation:

- Pull knee to chest, then pull knee and leg across body toward opposite shoulder to create stretch on outside of right hip.
- Hold easy stretch for 5–15 seconds.
- Do both sides.

Variation:

- From lying position, gently pull right knee toward outside of right shoulder.
- Hands should be placed on back of leg, just above knee.
- Hold 10–20 seconds.
- Breathe continuously and deeply.
- Repeat other leg.

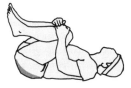

- After pulling one leg at a time to chest, pull both legs to chest.
- Concentrate on keeping back of head down, then curling head up toward knees.

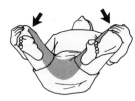

- Lie on back with knees flexed toward chest.
- Place hands on lower legs just below knees.
- Slowly pull legs out and down until you feel a mild stretch.
- Hold 10 seconds.
- The back of head can be flat on floor, resting on small pillow, or up off floor so you can look between legs.

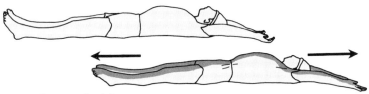

- Straighten out both legs again.
- Stretch and then relax.

A Stretch for the Lower Back and Side of Hip

- Lie on floor, legs straight.
- Bend left knee; extend left arm straight out from side.
- Use right hand to pull knee across body.
- Turn head toward left arm.
- Keep shoulders flat on floor, feet and ankles relaxed.
- Hold 10–20 seconds.
- Stretch both sides.

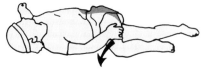

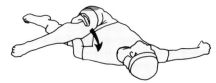

- To increase stretch in buttocks, reach under right leg and behind knee.
- Slowly pull right knee toward opposite shoulder until you get mild stretch.
- Keep both shoulders flat on floor.
- Hold 5–15 seconds.
- Do both legs.

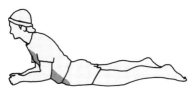

Back Extension:

- Start from prone position (lying on stomach).
- Place elbows beneath shoulders. Mild tension should be felt in middle to lower back area.
- Keep front of hips on floor.
- Hold 5–10 seconds.
- Repeat 2–3 times.

End series of back stretches by lying in fetal position.

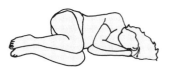

- Lie on side with legs curled up and head resting on hands.
- Relax.

SUMMARY OF STRETCHES FOR YOUR BACK

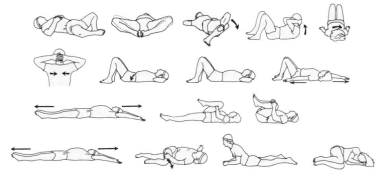

Do these stretches, in this order, to relax your back.

Learn to listen to your body. If the stretch builds or you feel pain, your body is trying to let you know that something is wrong, that there is a problem. If this happens, ease off gradually until the stretch feels right.

Stretches for the Legs, Feet, and Ankles

- Rotate ankle clockwise and counterclockwise through a complete range of motion with slight resistance provided by hand.
- This rotary motion helps to gently stretch out tight ankle ligaments.
- Repeat 10–20 times in each direction.
- Do both ankles.

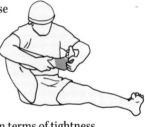

Feel if there is any difference between ankles in terms of tightness and range of motion. Sometimes ankle that has been sprained will feel weaker and tighter. Difference may go unnoticed until you work each ankle separately and make comparison.

- Next, use fingers to gently pull toes toward you to stretch top of foot and tendons of toes.
- Hold easy stretch 10 seconds.
- Repeat 2–3 times.
- Do both feet.
- Holding this position also helps relax bottom of foot *(plantar fascia).*

- Place thumbs at base of large toes (bottom of feet where toes come out of foot, index fingers slightly bent, and placed over nails of large toes.
- Use fingers and thumbs to move large toes back and forth 15–20 seconds.
- Rotate large toes in circular motion both clockwise and counterclockwise 10–15 seconds.
- Concentrate on increasing range of motion of toes as you manipulate area.
- Great way to improve or maintain the flexibility and circulation of area.

- With thumbs, massage up and down longitudinal arch of foot.
- Use circular motions with good amount of pressure to loosen tissues.
- Do both feet.
- Should help reduce tension and tightness in feet.

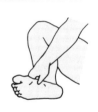

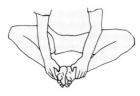

Variation:
- Massage arches of feet with thumbs.
- Move up and down arches, working out sore areas with circular massage.
- Good to do while watching TV or just before going to sleep.
- Massage with pressure that feels good.

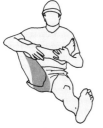

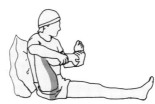

- Sit on floor with left leg straight out in front.
- Hold outside of right ankle with left hand, with right hand and forearm around bent knee.
- Gently pull leg *as one unit* toward chest until you feel easy stretch in back of upper leg; no stress at knee.
- You may rest back against something for support.
- Hold 10–20 seconds. Repeat other side.

For some of you, this position will not provide a stretch. If that is the case, do the stretch shown below.

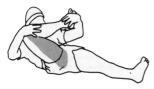

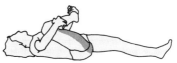

- Begin by lying down, then lean forward to hold onto leg as described in previous stretch.
- Gently pull leg as one unit toward chest until you feel easy stretch in butt and upper hamstring.

- Hold for 5–15 seconds.
- Doing stretch in lying position will increase stretch in hamstrings for people who are relatively flexible in area.
- Do both legs and compare.

Experiment:

See the difference in stretch when your head is forward and when back of head is on floor. Always keep every stretch within personal comfort range. Place small pillow behind head for comfort.

- Lie on back. Bend right knee and put outside of right lower leg just above opposite knee.
- With hands just below left knee, gently pull leg toward chest until stretch is felt in buttocks area *(piriformis)*.
- Hold 10–20 seconds. Stretch both legs.
- Lift back of head off floor and look straight ahead as you stretch.
- Breathe slowly and deeply.

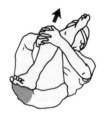

PNF Technique: *Contract — Relax — Stretch.*
- Another way to stretch buttocks is to use contract-relax-stretch technique.
- Starting from previous position, move left leg downward as you resist movement (contraction) for 4–5 seconds.
- Relax and stretch for 10–20 seconds as previously described.
- Really good stretch for *piriformis*.

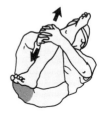

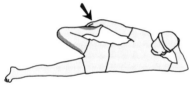

- Lie on left side.
- Rest side of head in palm of left hand.
- Hold top of right foot with your right hand between toes and ankle joint.
- Gently pull right heel toward right buttock to stretch ankle and quadriceps (front of thigh).
- Hold easy stretch 10 seconds.

Never stretch the knee to the point of pain. Always be in control.

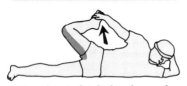

- Move front of right hip forward by contracting right thigh *(quadriceps)* muscles as you push right foot into right hand.
- Should stretch front of thigh and relax hamstrings.

- Hold easy stretch 10 seconds.
- Keep body in straight line.
- Now stretch left leg in the same way. (You may also get good stretch in front of shoulder.)

I like to follow this stretch with the hamstrings stretch at the top of page 58.

Stretching Your Iliotibial Bands

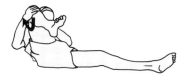

If you experience any knee pain with these stretches, don't do them. Instead, use the opposite-hand-to-opposite-foot technique of stretching the knee (p. 75).

- Lie on side while holding front of lower leg from outside with right hand.

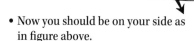

- Circle leg in front of you, then lightly behind you.
- As you circle leg, move right hand to top of right ankle.

- Now you should be on your side as in figure above.
- To stretch iliotibial band, gently pull right heel toward buttocks as

you move inside of your knee downward toward floor.
- You should feel stretch on outside of upper leg.
- Hold 10–15 seconds. Do both legs.

A Sitting Stretch for the Quadriceps:

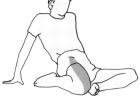

- Sit with right leg bent, with right heel just outside right hip.
- Left leg is bent and sole of left foot is next to inside of upper right leg.
- You can also do this stretch with left leg straight out in front of you.

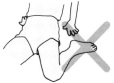

- Your foot should be extended back with ankle flexed.
- If ankle is too tight, move foot just enough to side to lessen tension in ankle.

- Do not let foot flare out to side in this position.
- By keeping foot pointed straight back, you take stress off inside of knee.
- More foot flares to side, more stress there is on knee.

- Now, slowly lean *straight back* until you feel easy stretch.
- Use hands for balance and support.
- Hold easy stretch 5–15 seconds.

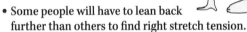

- Some people will have to lean back further than others to find right stretch tension.
- Some people may feel right stretch without leaning back at all.
- Be aware of how you feel and forget about how far you can go.
- Stretch to where you are comfortable and don't worry about anyone else.
- Do not let knee lift off floor or mat.

> Be sure to hold only stretches that are comfortable.
> **Be careful not to overstretch.**

- Now slowly, and in complete control and comfort, increase into developmental stretch.
- Hold 10 seconds, slowly come out of it.
- Switch sides and stretch left thigh same way.
- Can you feel any difference in tension? Is one side more limber than the other? Are you more flexible on one side?

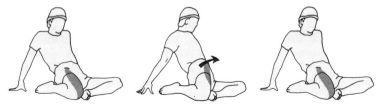

- After stretching quads, practice tightening buttocks on side of bent leg as you turn hip over.
- After contracting butt *(gluteus)* muscles 5–8 seconds, let buttocks relax.
- Drop hip down and continue to stretch quads another 10–15 seconds.
- Practice to eventually get both sides of buttocks to touch floor at same time during stretch.
- Do other side.

Note: Stretching the quads first, then turning the hip over as the buttocks contract will help change the stretch feeling when you return to the original quads stretch.

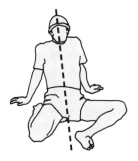

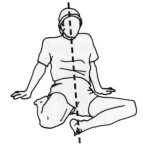

- If this produces pain in knee, move knee of leg being stretched closer to midline of body until it's more comfortable.
- Moving this way may take stress off knee, but if there is continuing pain, stop doing this stretch.

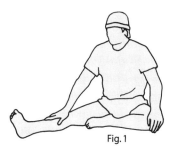

Fig. 1

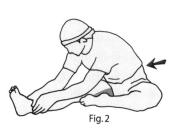

Fig. 2

- Sit on floor, legs straight out at sides.
- Bend left leg in at knee *(fig. 1)*.
- Slowly bend forward from hips toward foot of straight leg until you feel slight stretch *(fig. 2)*.
- Do not dip head forward at start of stretch.
- Hold developmental stretch 10–20 seconds.
- Repeat other side.
- Foot of straight leg upright, ankles and toes relaxed.
- Use a towel if you cannot easily reach feet.

I have found that it is best to stretch your quads first, then the hamstrings of the same leg. It is easier to stretch the hamstrings after the quadriceps have been stretched.

Use a towel or elastic cord to help you stretch if you cannot *easily* reach your foot.

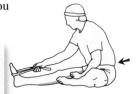

Get used to doing variations of basic stretches. In each variation you will use your body in a different way. You will become more aware of all the stretch possibilities when you change the angles of the stretch tension, even if the angle changes are very slight.

Variations of the Straight-leg, Bent-knee Position

- Reach across body with left arm to outside of right leg.
- Place right hand out to side for balance. This will stretch the muscles of upper back and spine and side of lower back, as well as hamstrings.
- To change stretch, look over right shoulder as you turn front of left hip slightly to inside.
- Breathe easily. Do not hold breath.
- Hold 10–15 seconds.

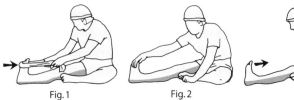

| Fig. 1 | Fig. 2 | Fig. 3 |

- To stretch back of lower leg, use towel around ball of foot to pull toes toward knee *(fig. 1)*.
- Or if you are more flexible, use hand to pull toes toward knee *(fig. 2)*.

- Or pull foot toward knee (dorsiflexion) without using hand, and hold, then lean slightly forward to stretch calf *(fig. 3)*.
- Hold 10–20 seconds.

PNF Technique: Contract — Relax — Stretch.

- Another way to stretch back of lower leg is to first contract area by pushing foot downward as you resist with towel for 4–5 seconds. Then relax.
- Now use towel to pull foot toward knee.
- Hold 5–15 seconds.

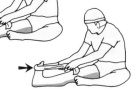

- To stretch outside of lower leg, reach down with opposite hand and hold outside border of foot *(see drawing)*.
- Now, gently turn outside of foot to inside to feel stretch on outside of lower leg.
- Stretch can be done with straight leg, or it can be done with leg flexed at knee if you are unable to *easily* hold outside border of foot with leg straight.
- In straight-leg position quadriceps should be soft and relaxed.
- Hold easy stretch 10 seconds.

Never lock your knees when doing sitting stretches. Be sure to keep the front of your thigh *(quadriceps)* relaxed in all positions using a straight leg. You can't stretch the hamstrings correctly when the opposing set of muscles (the quadriceps) are not relaxed.

SUMMARY OF STRETCHES FOR THE LEGS, FEET, AND ANKLES

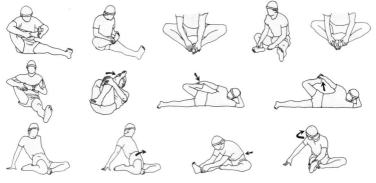

Do these stretches, in this order, as a routine.

Bouncing while stretching can actually make you tighter, rather than more flexible. For example, if you bounce four or five times while touching your toes, then bend over again several minutes later, you'll probably find that you are farther away from your toes than when you started! Each bouncing movement activates the stretch reflex, tightening the very muscles you are trying to stretch.

Stretches for the Back, Shoulders, and Arms

There are many stretches that can reduce tension and increase flexibility in the upper body. Most of the sitting or standing stretches can be done anywhere.

Many people suffer from tension in the upper body because of stress in their lives. Quite a few muscular athletes are stiff in the upper body because of not stretching that area.

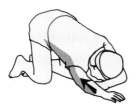 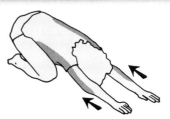

- Kneel with legs bent beneath you, rest forehead on left arm, and reach right arm forward.

- Pull back at hips, pressing palms down.
- Hold 10–20 seconds.
- Repeat on other side.

You can do this stretch one arm at a time or both at same time.

- Pulling with just one arm provides more control and isolates stretch on either side.

- By slightly moving your hips in either direction, you can increase or decrease stretch.
- Don't strain. Be relaxed. Hold 15 seconds.

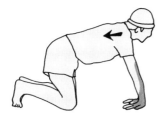

A Forearm and Wrist Stretch:

- Kneel on all fours with thumbs pointed out, fingers pointed toward knees.
- Palms flat, gently lean back.
- Hold 5–15 seconds, relax and repeat.

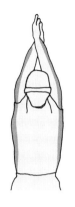

- With arms extended overhead and palms together, stretch arms upward and slightly backward.
- Breathe in as you stretch upward. Hold for 5–8 seconds. Breathe easily.

This is a great stretch for muscles of outer portions of arms, shoulders, and ribs. It can be done any time and any place to relieve tension and create feeling of relaxation and well-being.

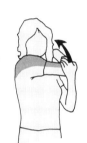

- With left hand, pull right elbow across chest toward left shoulder and hold 10 seconds.
- Repeat on other side.

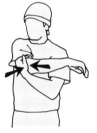
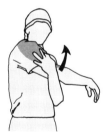

Fig. 1   Fig. 2

PNF Technique: *Contract — Relax — Stretch.*

- Stand with knees slightly flexed.
- With left hand, hold outside of right arm just above elbow.
- Move right arm away from body as you resist with left hand.
- Hold isometric contraction for 3–4 seconds *(fig. 1)*.
- After momentarily relaxing, gently pull arm across body toward shoulder until you feel a comfortable stretch in outside of shoulder and upper arm *(fig. 2)*.
- Hold 10 seconds, then repeat other side.

Here is a simple stretch for your triceps and the top of your shoulders.

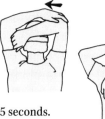

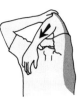

- With arms overhead, hold elbow of right arm with left hand.
- With left hand, pull right elbow across chest toward left shoulder and hold 10–15 seconds.
- Repeat other side.

PNF Technique: *Contract — Relax — Stretch.*

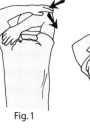

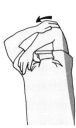

- Stand with knees slightly flexed and feet about shoulder-width apart.
- Hold right elbow with left hand.
- Move right elbow downward as you resist this movement with left hand (isometric contraction) 3–4 seconds *(fig.1).*
- After momentarily relaxing, gently pull elbow over, behind head until you feel mild stretch in back of upper arm *(fig.2).*
- Hold 5–15 seconds. Repeat other side.

Fig. 1

Fig. 2

- Stand or sit with arms overhead, knees slightly flexed.
- Hold elbow with hand of opposite arm.
- Pull elbow behind head gently as you slowly lean to side until mild stretch is felt.
- Hold 10–15 seconds.
- Repeat other side.

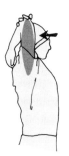

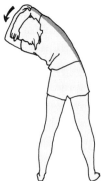

Variation:

- From standing position, knees slightly bent (1″), gently pull elbow behind head as you bend from hips to side.
- Hold easy stretch 10 seconds.
- Do both sides.
- *Keep knees slightly bent for better balance.*
- Do not hold breath.

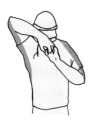

Another Shoulder Stretch:

- Reach behind head and down as far as you can with left hand.
- If you are able, grab right hand coming up, palm out.
- Grab your fingers and hold for 5–10 seconds.

If hands do not meet, try one of following:

- Have someone pull hands slowly toward each other until you get easy stretch and hold it.
- Do not stretch too far. You may get great stretch without touching fingers.

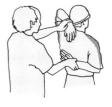

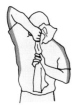

- Or drop a towel behind your head.
- With upper arm bent, reach up with other arm to hold onto end of towel.
- Gradually move hand up on towel, pulling upper arm downwards.

Work a little on it every day and get a good stretch. After a while you will be able to do this stretch without help. It reduces tension and increases flexibility. It also acts as an upper body revitalizer when you are tired.

- Interlace fingers out in front, palms out.
- Extend arms in front at shoulder height.
- Hold easy stretch 15 seconds.
- Relax, and repeat.

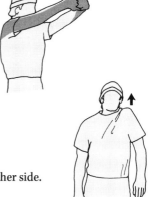

Single Shoulder Shrug:

- Start with shoulders relaxed downward.
- Bring left shoulder up toward left ear lobe.
- Hold for 3–5 seconds.
- Relax shoulder downward and repeat on other side.
- Excellent for shoulder tension.

PNF Technique: *Contract — Relax — Stretch.*

Shoulder Shrug:

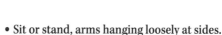

- Sit or stand with arms hanging loosely at sides.
- Shrug shoulders up.
- Hold 5 seconds.
- Relax shoulders downwards.

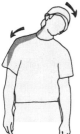

- Sit or stand, arms hanging loosely at sides.
- Tilt head sideways, first to one side, then the other.
- Keep shoulders relaxed downward during the stretch.
- Hold 5 seconds each side.

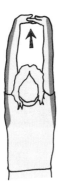

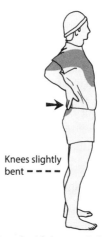

Knees slightly
bent − − − −

- Interlace fingers above head, palms upward.
- Push arms slightly back and up.
- Breathe easily.
- Hold 15 seconds.

- Stand with knees slightly flexed and place hands just above back of hips, elbows back.
- Gently press palms forward.
- Hold 10 seconds; repeat twice.
- Breathe easily.
- Keep knees flexed.
- Do this stretch after sitting for a long time.

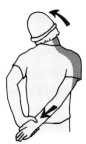

- Lean head sideways toward left shoulder.
- With left hand, gently pull right arm down and across, behind back.
- Hold 5–10 seconds.
- Repeat on other side.

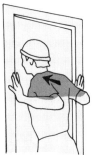

- Place hands shoulder height on either side of doorway.
- Move upper body forward until you feel comfortable stretch in arms, chest.
- Keep chest and head up, knees slightly bent.
- Hold 15 seconds.
- Breathe easily.

The next stretches are done with your fingers interlaced behind your back.

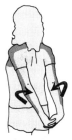

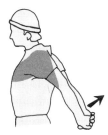

- Interlace fingers behind back, palms facing back.
- Slowly turn elbows inward while straightening arms until you feel stretch.
- Lift breast bone slightly upward as you stretch.
- Hold 5–10 seconds.

- If that is fairly easy, then lift arms up behind you until you feel stretch in arms, shoulders, or chest.
- Hold easy stretch for 5–10 seconds.
- Good to do when you find yourself slumping forward from shoulders.
- Keep chest out and chin in.
- Can be done any time.

SUMMARY OF STRETCHES FOR BACK, SHOULDERS, AND ARMS

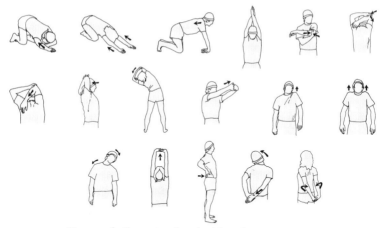

You can do these stretches, in this order, as a routine.

It is better to understretch than to overstretch. Always be at a point where you can stretch further, and never at a point where you have gone as far as you can go.

A Series of Stretches for the Legs

Toe Pointer: This is another good stretch for the legs. You can do a series of stretches for the legs, feet, and groin from the toe pointer position.

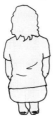

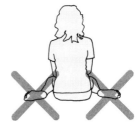

- This position helps stretch knees, ankles, and quadriceps.
- Toe pointing will help relax calves so they may be stretched more easily.

- Do not let feet flare out to sides when doing this stretch.

Note: A flared-out position of lower legs and feet may cause overstretching of inside *(medial collateral)* ligaments of knee.

Caution: If you have or have had knee problems, be very careful bending the knees underneath you. Do it slowly and under control. If there is any pain, discontinue the stretch.

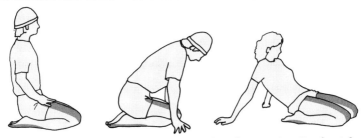

- Most women will not feel much of a stretch in this position. But for tight people, especially men, this position lets you know if you have tight ankles.
- If there is strain, place hands on outside of legs for support as you balance yourself slightly forward.
- Find position you can hold 10–30 seconds.

If you are tight, do not overstretch. Regularity in stretching creates positive change. There will be noticeable improvement in ankle flexibility within several weeks.

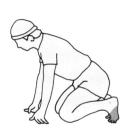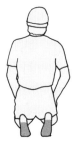

Variation:

- To stretch toes and bottom of foot *(plantar fascia)*, sit with toes underneath you.
- Put hands in front of you for balance and control.
- If you want to stretch further, slowly lean backwards until it feels right.
- Stretch easily 5–10 seconds.
- Be careful. There may be a lot of tension in this part of the foot and toes.
- Be patient. Gradually get body used to changing by stretching regularly.
- Return to toe pointer after doing this stretch.

To Stretch the Achilles Tendon Area and Ankles

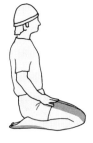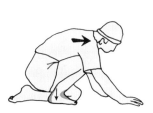

- Bring toes of one foot almost even with or parallel to knee of other leg.
- Let heel of bent leg come off ground one-half inch or so.
- Lower heel toward ground while leaning forward on thigh (just above knee) with chest and shoulder.
- The idea is not to get heel flat, but to use forward pressure from shoulder on thigh to gently stretch Achilles tendon area.
- Be careful. The Achilles tendon area needs only a *very slight stretch.*
- Hold 5–10 seconds; do other side.

This stretch is great for tight ankles and arches. Be sure to work both sides.

As we get older or go through periods of inactivity and then are active again, there is a lot of stress and strain on the lower legs, ankles, and arches. One way to reduce or eliminate the pain and soreness of new activity is to stretch before and after exercise.

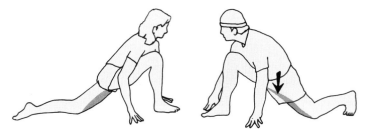

- Move one leg forward until knee of forward leg is directly over ankle.
- Place knee of other leg behind, resting on floor.
- Lower front of hip directly downward to create easy stretch.
- Hold 10–20 seconds.
- Repeat on other side.

Be careful if you have had knee problems. Do not stretch with any feeling of actual pain. Use control so you find the proper stretch feeling.

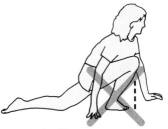

- *Do not have knee forward of ankle.*
- This will hinder proper stretching of hip and legs.
- The greater distance there is between back knee and heel of front foot, the easier it is to stretch hips and legs.

Stretching for 10–20 minutes in the evening is a good way to keep your muscles well tuned, so you feel good the next morning. If you have any tight areas, or soreness, stretch these areas before retiring (or while watching TV) and feel for yourself the difference the next morning.

Variations:

- Turn left hip slowly to inside to change area of stretch. By only slightly changing angles, you are able to stretch many different, adjacent areas of body.
- Hold easy stretch 5–15 seconds.
- Stretch both legs.
- This is excellent for hips, lower back, and groin.
- Look over your shoulder, behind you, to stretch neck and upper back.

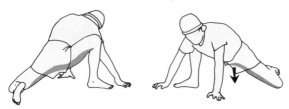

- From previous hip stretch, bend rear knee and move rear foot to inside, making 90° angle at knee joint.
- Move shoulders off knee and put hands to inside of body for support.
- Move hips downward to stretch inside of upper leg (groin).
- Do not move back knee or front foot.
- Be sure that front knee is directly above ankle.
- Hold easy stretch 5–15 seconds. Now do other side.

An excellent stretch for hip flexibility:

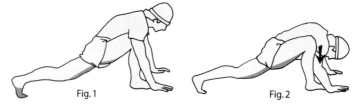

Fig. 1   Fig. 2

- With front knee directly above ankle, shift weight up onto toes and ball of back foot *(fig. 1)*.
- Hold easy stretch with fairly straight back leg 15–20 seconds.
- Think of front of hip going down to create right stretch tension.
- Use hands for balance. Do both legs.
- Another variation is to change stretch by gently lowering upper body to inside of knee of forward leg *(fig. 2)*.
- Hold comfortable stretch 10–15 seconds.

Also, you can stretch your pelvic area with your upper body upright as shown in the next two stretches.

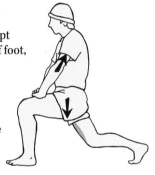

- Start with one leg in front of other, with ankle of front leg directly below your front knee. Other knee is resting on floor.
- Place hands on top of each other on thigh, just above knee.
- To stretch front of hip and thigh, straighten arms to keep upper body upright, as you lower front of hip downward. This is an excellent stretch for front of hip *(iliopsoas)* and good for lower back area.
- Hold 5–15 seconds. Repeat other side.

- Use same technique as in last stretch, except back knee is off floor and you are on ball of foot, making back leg much straighter.
- This stretch further promotes flexibility in pelvis/hip area. Hold 5–15 seconds.
- Do both sides.
- This position will challenge you to balance and stretch at same time. As in previous stretch, lower front of hip downward as you keep torso upright (vertical).

SUMMARY OF STRETCHES FOR LEGS

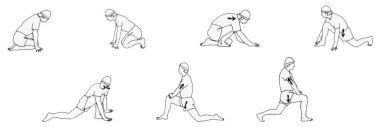

Do these leg stretches, in this order, as a routine.

Stretches for the Lower Back, Hips, Groin, and Hamstrings

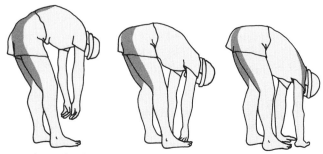

- Feet about shoulder-width apart and pointed straight ahead.
- Slowly bend forward from hips.
- *Keep knees slightly bent* (1″) during stretch so lower back is not stressed. Let neck and arms relax.
- Go to point where you feel slight stretch in back of legs.
- Stretch for 5–15 seconds, until you are relaxed. Mentally concentrate on area being stretched.
- Do not lock knees or or bounce. Simply hold an easy stretch.

When you do this stretch, you will feel it mostly in your hamstrings (back of thighs) and back of the knees. Your back will also be stretched, but you will feel this stretch mostly in the back of your legs.

> Stretch by how you *feel* and not by how *far* you can go.

Coming Back to an Upright Position

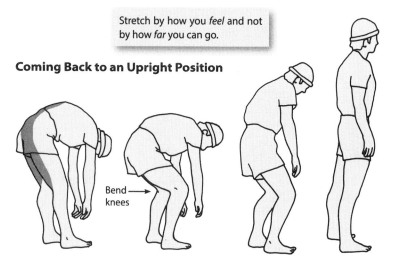

Bend → knees

Important:

- Whenever you bend at waist to stretch, remember to bend knees slightly (1″ or so). It takes pressure off lower back.
- Use big muscles of upper legs to stand up, instead of small muscles of lower back.
- Never bring yourself to upright position with knees locked.

Stretching is not competitive. You may well not be able to touch your toes. The point is for *you* to get more flexible, not to stretch as far as others.

This principle is also important in lifting heavy objects off ground. (*See pp. 232–234*, Caring for Your Back.)

PNF Technique: *Contract — Relax — Stretch.*

- Stand with feet shoulder-width apart.
- Bend knees, heels flat, toes pointed straight ahead.
- Hold 30 seconds.

In this bent-knee position, you are contracting the quadriceps and relaxing the hamstrings. The primary function of the quadriceps is to straighten the leg. The basic function of the hamstrings is to bend the knee. Because these muscles have opposing actions, contracting the quadriceps will relax the hamstrings.

As you hold this bent-knee position, feel the difference between the front and the back of your thigh. The quadriceps should feel hard and tight, while the hamstrings should feel soft and relaxed. It's easier to stretch the hamstrings if they are first relaxed.

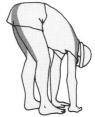

 quadriceps   hamstrings

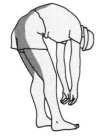 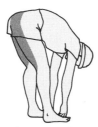

- After holding bent-knee position, stand up and then bend down again with knees slightly bent (1″).
- Don't bounce. You probably can go a little farther already.
- Hold about 5–15 seconds.

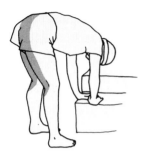

- Stand with feet shoulder width apart, heels flat, toes pointed straight ahead.
- With knees slightly bent, bend forward at hips; arms and neck relaxed.
- If you can't reach toes or ankles, use a stair, curb, or pile of books to rest hands on.
- Hold 10–20 seconds.
- Do not lock knees or bounce.
- Keep knees slightly bent as you return to upright position.

Variation:

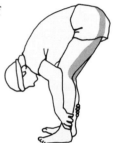

- With hands, hold onto back of lower legs in calf or ankle area.
- By pulling upper body downward (gently!) with hands, you will be able to increase the stretch in legs and back, while you concentrate on relaxing in a very stable position.
- Do not go too far.
- Relax and stretch.
- Knees slightly bent.

Always remember to bend your knees when standing up. This lessens any strain on the lower back.

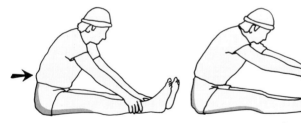

- Sit with legs straight and feet upright, heels no more than 6″ apart.
- Bend from hips to get easy stretch.
- Hold 5–15 seconds.
- You will probably feel this just behind knees and in back of upper legs.
- You may also feel stretch in lower back if back is tight.

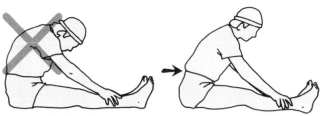

- Do not dip head forward as you begin this stretch.
- Try to keep hips from rolling backwards.

- Think of bending from hips without rounding upper back.

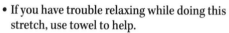

- You may need to sit against wall to keep lower back flat.
- This position in itself may be enough of a stretch for you if you are extremely tight.

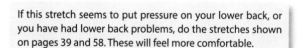

- If you have trouble relaxing while doing this stretch, use towel to help.
- Pull yourself forward (gently!) from hips to where you can relax and still stretch.
- Use hands and arms to pull yourself forward.
- Work down the towel with fingers, until stretch feels right.
- Be careful here. Do not overstretch.

> If this stretch seems to put pressure on your lower back, or you have had lower back problems, do the stretches shown on pages 39 and 58. These will feel more comfortable.

- Be careful when you stretch with both legs in front of you or when bending forward at hips in standing position.
- You must not overstretch in these positions. Each leg differs in tightness, so don't stretch both legs at same time if you have lower back problems.
- When one or both legs are extremely tight, it's difficult to stretch both legs at the same time and get correct stretch for each leg.
- It is easier on back to stretch each leg separately.

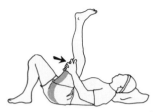

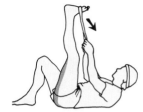

- Lie on back and lift leg up toward 90° angle at thigh joint.
- Keep lower back flat against floor.
- Hold 10–20 seconds. Repeat for other leg.

- If necessary, hold onto back of leg to create stretch, or put towel around bottom of foot and pull gently.
- Place pillow under head for more comfort.

To Stretch the Groin Area

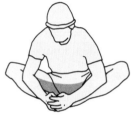

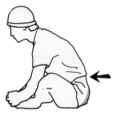

- Sit on floor, soles of feet together, holding onto toes and feet.
- Gently pull forward, bending from hips.

- Hold 10–30 seconds.
- Do not bounce.
- Breathe slowly and deeply.

> Remember — no bouncing when you stretch. Find a place that is fairly comfortable, one that allows you to stretch and relax at the same time.

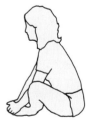

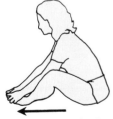

If you have any trouble bending forward, your heels may be too close to your groin area.

If so, move your feet farther out in front of you. This will allow you to move forward from your hips.

Variations If You Are Tight in the Groin Area

- Hold onto feet with one hand, with elbow on inside of lower leg to hold down and stabilize leg.
- With other hand on inside of your leg *(not on knee)*, gently push leg downward to isolate and stretch this side of groin.
- If you are tight in groin area, this is a good isolation stretch that will allow knees to fall more naturally downward.
- Do both sides. Hold 10–15 seconds.

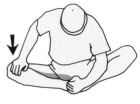

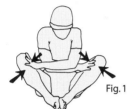

Fig. 1

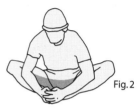

Fig. 2

PNF Technique: *Contract — Relax — Stretch.*

- With hands supplying slight resistance on insides of opposite thighs, try to bring knees together just enough to contract muscles in groin *(fig. 1)*.
- Hold 4–5 seconds, then relax and stretch groin as in preceding stretches *(fig. 2)*.

This contract-relax stretch will help relax a tight groin area.

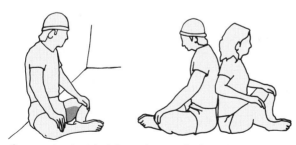

Another way to stretch tight groin muscles is to sit against a wall or something else for support.

- Back straight, soles of feet together, use hands to push gently down on inside of thighs (not *on* knees, just above them).
- Push gently until you get a good, even stretch. Relax and hold 20–30 seconds.

It is also possible to do this stretch with a partner. Sit back-to-back for stability.

If you have trouble sitting cross-legged, these groin stretches will start to make that position easier for you.

- To stretch back and inside of legs, sit in crossed-leg position and then lean forward until you feel a good comfortable stretch.
- Get elbows out in front of you if you can.
- Hold and relax.
- This is a simple stretch for most people and feels good in lower back.
- Do not hold breath.
- Stretch 15–20 seconds.

Variation:

- Move upper body over knee instead of straight ahead. This is good for hips.
- Think of bending from hips.

The Spinal Twist

The spinal twist is good for the upper back, lower back, side of hips, and rib cage. It will improve your ability to turn to the side or look behind you without having to turn your entire body.

- Sit on floor, right leg straight out in front.
- Bend left leg, cross left foot over, place outside right knee.
- Bend right elbow and rest it outside left knee.
- Place left hand behind hips on floor.
- Turn head over left shoulder, rotate upper body left.
- Hold 10–15 seconds.
- Repeat on other side.
- Breathe slowly.
- Left arm behind you, turn and look over left shoulder.
- Rotate upper body to left; think of turning hips at same time (although they won't move).
- This stretches lower back and side of hip.
- Hold 5–15 seconds.
- Do both sides.

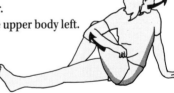

Breathing:
- Deep
- Relaxed
- Rhythmic

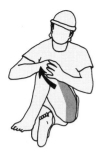

Variation:

- Sit on floor with right leg straight out in front.
- Bend left leg, cross left foot over, place outside right knee.
- Pull left knee across body toward opposite shoulder.
- Hold 10–15 seconds.
- Repeat on other side.
- Breathe easily.

People tend to spend more time on the first leg, arm, or area they stretch, and they usually will stretch their "easy" or more flexible side first. Thus more time is spent on the "good" side and less on the "bad" side. To remedy this, stretch your tight side first. This will help even out your overall flexibility.

SUMMARY OF STRETCHES FOR LOWER BACK, HIPS, GROIN, AND HAMSTRINGS

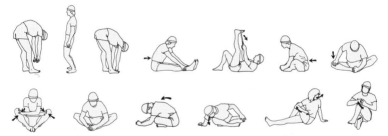

You can do these stretches, in this order, as a routine.

At this time let's go over some of the basic techniques of stretching:

- Don't stretch too far, especially in the beginning. Get a slight stretch and increase it after you feel yourself relax.

- Hold a stretch in a comfortable position; the stretch tension should subside as you hold it. No drastic static stretches.

- Breathe slowly, deeply, and naturally — exhale as you bend forward. Do not stretch to a point where you cannot breathe normally.

- Do not bounce. Bouncing tightens the very muscles you are trying to stretch.

- *Think about the area being stretched.* Feel the stretch. If the tension becomes greater as you stretch, you are overdoing it. Ease off into a more comfortable position.

- Don't focus on flexibility. Just learn to stretch properly and flexibility will come with time. (Flexibility is only one of the many by-products of stretching.)

Other things to be aware of:

- We are different every day. Some days we are tighter, other days looser.

- Drink plenty of water. Your muscles stretch more easily when your body is properly hydrated.

- You can control what you feel by what you do.

- Regularity is one of the most important factors in stretching. Stretch regularly and you will naturally want to become more active and fit.

- Don't compare yourself with others. Even if you are tight or inflexible, don't let this stop you from stretching and improving yourself.

- Proper stretching means stretching within your own limits, being relaxed, and not making comparisons with what other people can do.

- Stretching keeps your body ready for movement.

- Stretch whenever you feel like it. It will always make you feel good.

Stretches for the Back, Hips, and Legs

It's best to stretch on a firm but not hard surface, such as a soft rug or firm mat, when doing these stretches for the back. If the surface is too hard, you won't be able to relax as easily.

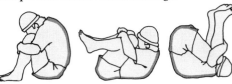

- Lie on back and pull left leg toward chest.
- Keep back of head on mat if possible, but don't strain.
- If you can't do it with head down, use small pillow under head.
- Keep other leg as straight as possible, without locking knee.
- Hold 30 seconds. Do both sides.
- This slowly loosens up back muscles and hamstrings.

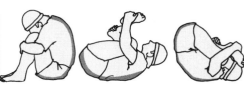

Spinal Roll:

- Don't do this stretch on a hard surface; use mat or rug.
- In sitting position hold knees with hands and pull to chest.
- Gently roll up and down your spine, keeping chin down toward chest. This further stretches muscles along spine.
- Roll back and forth 4–8 times or until you feel back start to limber up.
- Do not rush.

Remember: If you have a neck problem, be very careful with these stretches.

Spinal Roll with Crossed Legs:

- Begin roll in same sitting position as for previous spinal roll.
- As you roll backwards, cross lower legs and, at same time, pull feet (from the outside) toward chest.
- Release feet as you roll up to sitting position with feet together and uncrossed. (Always start each roll with legs uncrossed.)
- On each repetition, alternate crossing of lower legs so that, with pull-down phase of the roll, lower back will be stretched evenly on both sides.
- Do 6–8 repetitions.

Take your time in stretching your back. Do not rush through the stretches. Concentrate on relaxing in every stretch that you do. Find a stretch tension that feels good. Do not torture yourself.

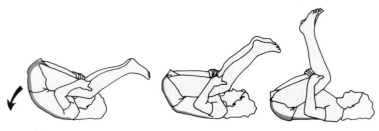

- With legs in moderate overhead position, roll down slowly, trying to lower each vertebra, one at a time. At first you will probably come down fast, but with practice, back will limber up so you can lower slowly, vertebra after vertebra.
- Put hands directly behind knees and *keep knees bent* as you roll down.
- Use arms and hands to hold legs still. This allows greater control of speed of downward roll.
- Keep head on floor. You may need to tilt head slightly upward for balance as you roll downward.

Rolling out of the legs-overhead position slowly like this is a good way to find out exactly what part of your back is the tightest. The parts of your back that are the hardest to lower *slowly* are the tightest. You can stretch tightness out of spine by working on it gently every day.

- To gain more control over stretch in back when lowering legs, place arms overhead and hold onto something that is stable such as a heavy piece of furniture.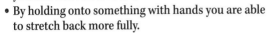
- Now, with slight bend in arms and bent knees, *slowly* lower yourself one vertebra at a time.
- By holding onto something with hands you are able to stretch back more fully.
- Do this slowly and under control.

> Do not overdo things, but instead, *gradually* develop your physical well-being.

Stretching with legs in a moderate overhead position is good for stretching the back and helps in the circulation of blood from the lower limbs to the upper body.

The Squat: Many of us get tired in the lower back from hours of standing and sitting. One position that helps to reduce this tension is the squat.

> **Be careful:** I believe that the squat is one of our most natural positions. However, due to particular knee problems, some people cannot and should not squat. Always check with a qualified professional if you have any concerns about what your body is capable of.

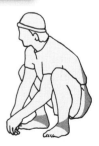

- From standing position, squat down with feet flat and toes pointed out at approximately 15° angles.
- Heels 4–12″ apart, depending on how limber you are, or as you become familiar with stretching, depending on exactly what parts of body you want to stretch.
- Squatting stretches knees, back, ankles, Achilles tendon areas, and deep groin. Keep knees to the outside of shoulders, directly above the big toes.
- Hold comfortably 10–15 seconds. For many people this will be easy, for others very difficult.

Variations: At first there may be a problem with balance, such as falling backwards because of tight ankles and tight Achilles tendons. If you are unable to squat as shown above, there are other ways to learn this position.

Try the squat on the downward slant of a driveway or hillside

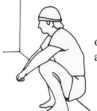

or by leaning your back against a wall.

You can use a fence or pole for balance.

After you have done it for a while, the squat becomes a very comfortable position and helps relieve tightness in the lower back. Now return to a standing position as shown on the opposite page.

Variations:

- From standing position, place hands slightly to inside of upper legs, just above knees.
- Keep feet shoulder-width apart.
- Slowly lower hips downward as you gently push upper legs outward until you feel mild stretch in groin area.
- Hold 15 seconds.
- This also stretches ankles and Achilles tendon area.
- Don't let hips drop below knees.

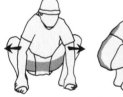
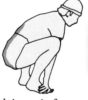

Be careful if you have had any knee problems. If pain is present, discontinue this stretch.

- To increase stretch in groin from squat position, put your elbows inside of knees and gently push outward with both elbows as you bend slightly forward from hips.
- Thumbs should be on inside of feet, with fingers along outside of feet.
- Hold 15 seconds. Do not overstretch.
- If you have trouble balancing, elevate heels slightly.

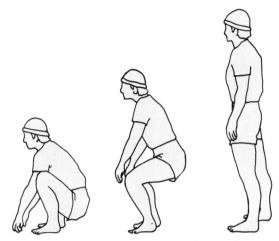

- To stand up from the squat position, pull your chin in slightly and rise straight up *with quadriceps doing all the work and back straight.*
- Do not dip head forward as you stand up; this puts too much pressure on lower back and neck.

SUMMARY OF STRETCHES FOR THE BACK, HIPS, AND LEGS

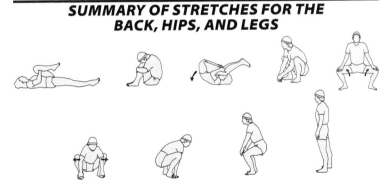

You can do these stretches, in this order, as a routine for your back.

Holding the right stretch tensions for a period of time allows the body to adapt to these new positions. Soon the area being stretched will adapt to the slight tension and your body will be able to assume the new positions without the tightness formerly felt.

Elevating Your Feet

Elevation of the feet before and after activity is a great way to revitalize your legs. It helps keep the legs light with plenty of consistent energy for everyday living and activity. It's a wonderful way to rest and relax tired feet, especially if you have been standing all day. It helps the entire body feel good. And it's a simple way to help prevent or relieve varicose veins. I recommend elevating the feet at least twice a day for 2–3 minutes or longer for revitalization and relaxation.

- Lying on the floor and resting feet against wall is simple way to elevate feet.
- Keep lower back flat, butt at least 3″ from wall.
- If there isn't a wall close by, you can elevate feet from legs-overhead position or simply put a few pillows under feet to raise them above heart.
- At first, elevate feet for only about 1 minute, gradually increasing time.
- If feet start to go to sleep, roll over on side and then sit up. (See p. 20 for the proper way to sit up from this position.)
- *Don't get up quickly after elevating feet or you may get a light-headed feeling.*

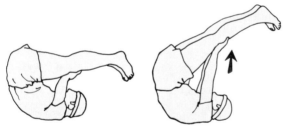

- Put palms of hands on knees with fingers pointed toward toes.
- Straighten arms.
- If you relax at the hips, arms will take care of weight of legs.
- This is a very relaxing position. In hatha yoga it is called the "pose of tranquility."
- There is a balancing point, at the back of head and top of spine when you are in this position.
- The balance is difficult to find but not as hard as it might seem at first. Give it at least 10–12 good tries. A little practice makes it simple.
- *Be careful doing this if you have any problem with upper back or neck.*

The BodySlant®:

- A great way to elevate your feet and stretch is to lie on a BodySlant.
- Don't do any exercises on the BodySlant; just lie there and relax for about 5 minutes, gradually increasing time to 15–20 minutes.
- Placing hands on chest or stomach will decrease arch in lower back.
- Good position for pulling in stomach and being thin. Internal organs will gradually fall back into normal position. For people who want to look and feel thin, the BodySlant is excellent.
- When getting up from the BodySlant, sit up for 2–3 minutes before you stand.
- Get up slowly from all positions with feet elevated so you don't become dizzy.

Stretching on the BodySlant

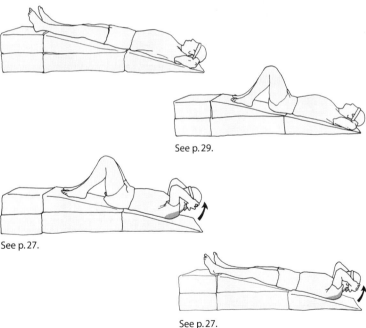

See p. 29.

See p. 27.

See p. 27.

We may know that stretching and regular exercising are beneficial, but knowledge alone is not enough. *Doing* is what is important, for what good is knowledge if we do not use it to live more fully?

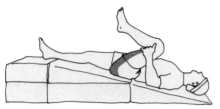

See p. 31.

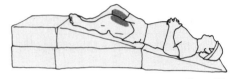

See p. 26.

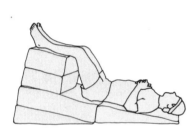

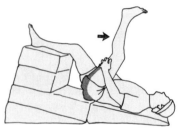

See p. 58.

SUMMARY OF STRETCHES FOR
ELEVATING YOUR FEET

   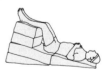

Standing Stretches for the Legs and Hips

This series of stretches will help your walking or running. It will give flexibility and energy to your legs. All these stretches can be done while standing.

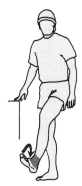

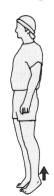

- Stand and hold onto something for balance.
- Lift right foot and rotate foot and ankle 8–10 times clockwise, then 8–10 times counterclockwise.
- Repeat on other side.

(**Note:** This can also be done sitting.)

PNF Technique: *Contract — Relax — Stretch.*

- Before stretching calves, stand on toes for 3–4 seconds to contract calves.
- Use following calf stretch to make it easier.

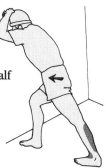

- Stand a little way from wall and lean on it with forearms, head resting on hands.
- Place right foot in front of you, leg bent, left leg straight behind you.
- Slowly move hips forward until you feel stretch in calf of left leg.
- Keep left heel flat and toes pointed straight ahead.
- Hold easy stretch 10–20 seconds.
- Do not bounce.
- Repeat on other side.
- Do not hold breath.

To create a stretch for the *soleus* and Achilles tendon area from the previous stretch:

- Lower hips downward.
- Slightly bend your left knee, keeping your back flat.
- Keep your left foot slightly toed-in or straight, heel down.
- Hold 10 seconds.
- Repeat other leg.

Note: The Achilles tendon area needs only a *slight feeling of stretch.*

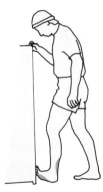

- The Achilles tendon area and ankle may be stretched another way.
- Place left foot against wall, ankle flexed and toes up.
- Move upper body forward until you feel mild stretch tension in Achilles tendon area.
- Hold 8–10 seconds.
- This also stretches the bottom of foot and toes.

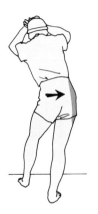

- To stretch outside of hip, start from same position as in calf stretch.
- Stretch right side of hip by turning right hip slightly to inside.
- Project side of right hip to side as you lean shoulders very slightly in opposite direction of hips.
- Hold an even stretch 5–15 seconds.
- Do both sides.
- Keep foot of back leg pointed straight ahead with heel flat on ground.

Lifelong Fitness Could Start in School

In the old days, high school students spent many hours in PE classes, learning only games and sports. If stretching was taught at all, it was the bouncing, "no pain — no gain" approach. These days a new generation of teachers has the opportunity to teach students how to take care of themselves: to stretch properly, to eat right, to make exercise a natural component of a healthy lifestyle. It would be great if kids could come out of school with a positive attitude toward staying healthy for the rest of their lives.

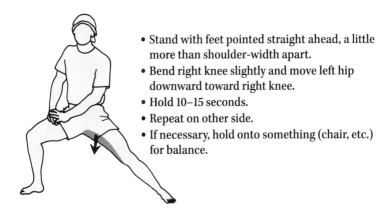

- Stand with feet pointed straight ahead, a little more than shoulder-width apart.
- Bend right knee slightly and move left hip downward toward right knee.
- Hold 10–15 seconds.
- Repeat on other side.
- If necessary, hold onto something (chair, etc.) for balance.

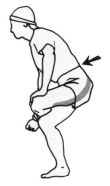

- Stand on one foot with knee slightly flexed and place outside of opposite leg just above knee.
- Put one hand on inside of ankle and other on thigh.
- Now bend knee a little more as you move chest forward over bent leg.
- This will test your balance.
- Hold mild stretch 5–10 seconds.
- Do both sides.
- This stretches outside of hip (*piriformis* area).
- Do not hold your breath.

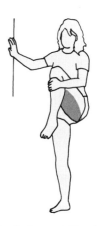

- Hold onto something and pull knee toward chest.
- Do not lean forward at waist or hips.
- This gently stretches upper hamstrings, butt, and hips.
- Foot on ground should be pointed straight ahead, with knee slightly bent (1″).
- Hold easy stretch 5–15 seconds.
- Do both legs.

- Place ball of foot up on secure support (wall, fence, table).
- Keep standing leg pointed straight ahead.
- Bend knee of raised leg as you move hips forward. This should stretch groin, hamstrings, and front of hip.
- Hold 10–15 seconds.
- Do both sides.
- If you can, for balance and control, use hands to hold onto support. This stretch will make it easier to lift knees.

Variation:

- Instead of having standing foot pointed straight ahead, turn it to side (parallel to support).
- Stretch inside of upper legs.
- Hold 10–15 seconds.

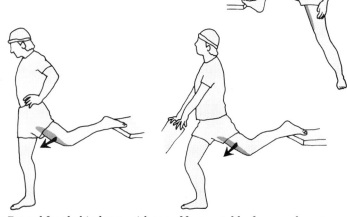

- Extend foot behind you, with top of foot on table, fence, or bar at comfortable height.
- Think of moving leg forward from front of hip to stretch front of hip and quadriceps. Flex butt *(gluteus)* muscles.
- Keep standing with knee slightly bent (1″), upper body vertical, foot on ground pointed straight ahead.
- Change stretch by slightly bending knee of supporting leg a little more.
- Hold an easy stretch 5–15 seconds.
- Through relaxed practice, learn to feel balanced and comfortable in this stretch.
- Breathe.
- Use chair or something for balance if necessary.

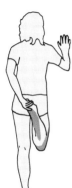

To stretch the quads and knee:

- Stand a little way from wall and place right hand on wall for support.
- Standing straight, grasp top of right foot with left hand.
- Pull heel toward buttock.
- Hold 10–20 seconds.
- Repeat on other side.

Variation:

- This stretch can also be done lying on stomach.
- Be sure to stretch without pain.
- Reach behind with hand and hold top of opposite foot between ankle joint and toes.
- Gently pull heel toward middle of buttocks.
- Hold 5–15 seconds.

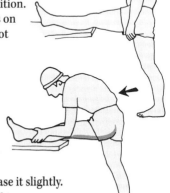

Important note: If you have knee problems, be very careful with these stretches.

- Place back of lower leg on table or ledge that is about waist-high or at comfortable height.
- Leg on ground should be slightly bent at knee (1″), with foot pointed forward as in proper running or walking position.
- Be careful to not overstretch in this position. Overstretching can put too much stress on back of knee, especially if lower leg is not supported fully.

Keep your knees slightly flexed with all these leg-up stretches.

- Now, while looking straight ahead, slowly bend forward at hips until you feel a good stretch in back of raised leg.
- Hold 5–15 seconds and relax.
- Find easy stretch, relax, and then increase it slightly.
- This is very good before running or walking.

Remember to stretch under control. Start in a place that is fairly easy and go from there. Improvement will occur faster if you go from an easy stretch to a developmental stretch. Let yourself limber up slowly. Remember, straining will keep you from fully realizing the many benefits of stretching.

- To stretch inside of raised leg, turn foot that is on the ground so it is parallel to support.
- Face upper body in the same direction as standing foot and turn right hip slightly to the inside.
- Slowly bend sideways with your right shoulder going toward right knee. This stretches the inside of upper right leg.
- Hold easy stretch for 5–15 seconds.
- Be sure to keep knee of standing leg slightly bent.
- Repeat for the other leg.

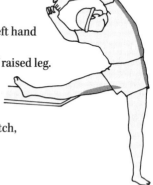

Variation:

- To change stretch, use right hand to pull left hand and arm up and over head.
- Good for sides of upper body and inside of raised leg.
- Keep knee of standing leg slightly bent.
- Hold easy stretch 5–15 seconds.
- Do both sides.
- Feel difference in each side. To do this stretch, you must be fairly flexible.

> **Remember:** Take care with these more difficult stretches, which require balance, strength, and a certain amount of flexibility.

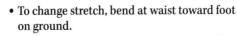

- To change stretch, bend at waist toward foot on ground.
- Raised leg should remain straight but will turn to inside as you bend over.
- This stretches hamstrings of supporting leg.
- Knee of that leg should be slightly bent (1″) during stretch.
- Hold easy stretch 5–15 seconds.
- Do not hold breath.

- If you want to stretch groin area of raised leg, bend knee of supporting leg and keep raised leg straight.
- If you can, rest hands on ground to give you added balance.
- Hold easy stretch 5–15 seconds.

SUMMARY OF STANDING STRETCHES
FOR THE LEGS AND HIPS

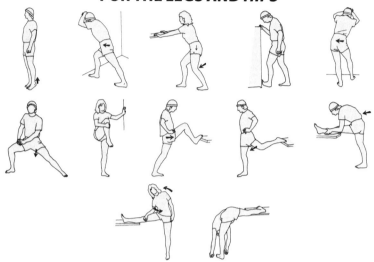

You can do these stretches, in this order, as a routine for the legs and hips.

Avoid creeping *rigor mortis*: It is important to maintain good flexibility throughout our lives, so that as we get older we can avoid the problems that go with stiff joints, tight muscles, and bad posture. One of the striking characteristics of aging is the loss of range of motion, and stretching is perhaps the single most important thing you can do to keep your body limber.

Standing Stretches for the Upper Body

These next two stretches are excellent for stretching the muscles along your side from your arm to your hips. They are done standing, so you can do them at any time, anywhere. Remember to keep your knees slightly bent (flexed) for better balance and to protect your lower back.

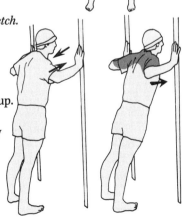

• Stand with feet about shoulder-width apart, toes pointed straight ahead.
• With knees slightly bent (1"), place one hand on hip for support while you extend other arm up and over head.
• Slowly bend at waist to side, toward hand on hip.
• Move slowly; feel a good stretch.
• Hold 5–15 seconds and relax.
• Gradually increase amount of time you are able to hold stretch.
• No quick or jerky movements; breathe and relax.

• Instead of using hand on hip for support, extend both arms overhead.
• Grasp right hand with left hand and bend slowly to left, using left arm to gently pull right arm over head and down toward ground.
• By using one arm to pull the other you can increase stretch along sides and along spine.
• *Do not overstretch.*
• Hold easy stretch 8–10 seconds.

PNF Technique: *Contract — Relax — Stretch.*

• Stand behind doorway with hands on door jambs a little above shoulder height.
• With arms bent, push yourself back by straightening arms, as in a push-up.
• Do 3–5 repetitions of this exercise, then relax and slowly let upper body go toward doorway to stretch front of shoulders and chest.
• Hold 15–20 seconds at comfortable tension.

This stretch for the upper body stretches the muscles laterally along the spine.

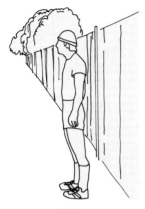

Fig. 1

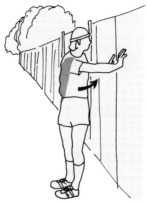

Fig. 2

- Stand about 12–24″ away from fence or wall with back toward it *(fig. 1)*.
- With feet about shoulder-width apart and toes pointed straight ahead, slowly turn upper body around until you can easily place hands on fence or wall at about shoulder height *(fig. 2)*.
- Turn in one direction and touch wall, return to starting position, and then turn in opposite direction and touch wall.

- Do not force yourself to turn any farther than is fairly comfortable.
- If you have knee problems, do this stretch very slowly and cautiously.
- Stop if there is pain. Be relaxed and do not overstretch.
- Hold 5–15 seconds.
- Keep knees slightly bent (1″).
- Do not hold breath.
- Stretch other side.

Variation:
- To change stretch, turn head and look over right shoulder.
- Try to keep hips facing forward and parallel to fence.
- Hold easy stretch 5–15 seconds.
- Do both sides.

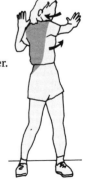

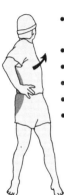

- Stand with hands on hips, feet straight ahead, knees slightly bent.
- Rotate hips to the left as you look over left shoulder.
- Hold 10–15 seconds.
- Repeat on other side.
- Keep knees slightly flexed.
- A good stretch for lower back, hips, and upper body.

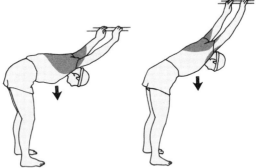

- Place both hands shoulder-width apart on a fence or ledge (or top of refrigerator or filing cabinet) and let upper body drop down as you keep knees slightly bent (1″).
- Keep hips directly above feet.
- Bend knees a bit more and feel stretch change.
- Place hands at different heights to change area of stretch.

- After you become familiar with this stretch it is possible to really stretch spine. Great to do if you have been slumping in upper back and shoulders all day. This will take some of the kinks out of tired upper back.
- Find stretch that you can hold for at least 20 seconds.
- Bend knees when coming out of stretch.

Variation:

- To increase and change area of stretch in another way, bring one leg behind and across midline of body as you lean in opposite direction.
- Will stretch hard-to-reach areas of upper body.
- Hold 10 seconds.
- Do both sides.

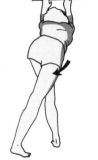

I find these arm and shoulder stretches to be very good before and after running. They allow for a relaxed upper body and a freer arm swing. They are also good to do during weight training workouts or as part of a warm-up for any upper body activity such as tennis, baseball, handball, etc.

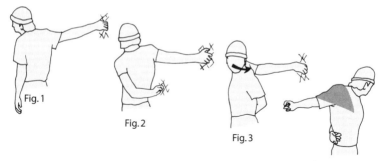

Fig. 1

Fig. 2

Fig. 3

View from the other side of the fence

- This stretch is for the front of shoulders and arms. You need a chain-linked fence, doorway, or wall.
- Face wall or press against it with right hand at shoulder level *(fig. 1)*.
- Bring other arm around back and grab wall (or whatever you are using) as in *fig. 2*.
- Look over left shoulder in direction of right hand.
- Keep shoulder close to wall as you slowly turn head *(fig. 3)*.
- Trying to look at right hand behind you gives you a stretch in front of shoulders.
- Stretch other side.
- Do it slowly and under control.

Variation:

- From previous position, stretch arm and shoulder at various angles.
- Each angle will stretch arm and shoulder differently.
- Hold 10 seconds.

Here is another stretch you can do while using a chain-linked fence or wall for support and balance.

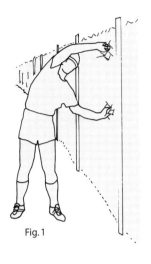

Fig. 1

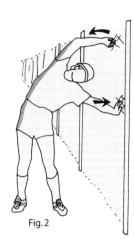

Fig. 2

- Hold onto fence at about waist-high with left hand.
- Now reach over your head with right arm and grab fence with right hand.
- Left arm will be slightly bent with right arm extended *(fig. 1)*.
- Keep knees slightly bent (1″).
- To stretch waistline and sides, straighten left arm and pull over with (upper) right arm *(fig. 2)*.
- Hold 5–10 seconds.
- Do both sides.

Slowly go into each stretch and slowly come out of each stretch. Do not bob, jerk, or bounce. Keep your stretching fluid and under control.

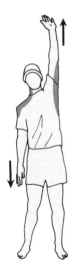

- Extend right arm above head.
- Reach down with left arm as you reach up with right arm.
- Point fingers.
- Hold 10 seconds.
- Repeat other side.
- If you do this stretch standing, keep knees slightly flexed.
- Breathe easily.

SUMMARY OF STANDING STRETCHES FOR THE UPPER BODY

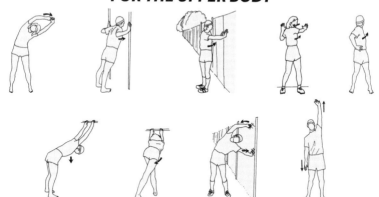

You can do these stretches, in this order, as a routine for the upper body.

Stretching on a Chin-up Bar

With the help of gravity, it is possible to get a fine stretch on a chin bar.

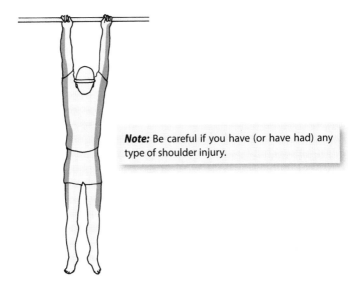

Note: Be careful if you have (or have had) any type of shoulder injury.

- Hold onto bar with both hands, relax chin forward as you hang, with feet off ground.
- A great stretch for upper body.
- Begin holding for 5 seconds, gradually increasing to at least 30 seconds.
- Strong grip will make stretch easier.

Enjoy stretching by the way it feels. If you torture yourself with drastic tensions in an attempt to get more flexible, you deprive yourself of the true benefits of stretching. If you stretch correctly, you'll find the more you stretch, the easier it becomes, and the easier you stretch, the more you will naturally enjoy it.

Stretches for the Upper Body Using a Towel

Most of us have a towel in our hands at least once a day. A towel or elastic cord can aid in stretching the arms, shoulders, and chest.

- Hold towel near both ends so that you can move it, with straight arms, up and over head and down behind back.
- Do not strain or force it.
- Hands should be far enough apart to allow for relatively free movement up and over head and down behind back.
- Breathe slowly.
- Do not hold breath.

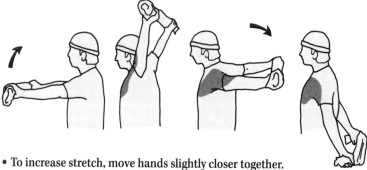

- To increase stretch, move hands slightly closer together.
- Keeping arms straight, repeat movement.
- Move slowly and feel stretch.
- Do not overstretch.
- If you are unable to go through full movement of up, over, and behind while keeping arms straight, then hands are too close together. Move them farther apart.
- You can hold stretch at any place during this movement. This will isolate and add more of a stretch to muscles of that particular area.
- For example, if chest is tight and sore, it is possible to isolate stretch there by holding towel at shoulder level with arms straight behind you, as shown above.
- Hold 5–15 seconds.

Stretching is not a contest. You needn't compare yourself with others, because we are all different. Moreover, each day we are different: some days we are more limber than others. Stretch comfortably, within your limits, and you will begin to feel the flow of energy that comes from proper stretching.

Here is another series of stretches using a towel.

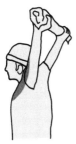

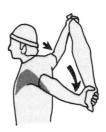

- Bring towel overhead, keeping arms straight.

- Lower left arm back and behind you at shoulder level as right arm bends to approximately a 90° angle.

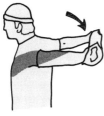

- Now straighten right arm out to same level as left arm and then simultaneously move both arms downward.
- This can be done slowly, in one complete movement, or you can stop at any point to increase stretch in that particular area.
- Do this completed movement toward other side by lowering right arm first.
- As you become more flexible, you will be able to hold towel with hands closer together. Do not strain.

I think that limberness in the shoulders and arms really helps tennis, running, walking, and of course swimming (to name only a few activities for which you need this flexibility). Stretching the chest area reduces muscle tension and tightness and increases circulation and ease of breathing. It is actually very simple to stretch and keep the upper body limber, if you do it *regularly*.

Note: Be careful if you have (or have had) any type of shoulder injury. Proceed slowly and discontinue if there is pain.

A Series of Stretches for the Hands, Wrists, and Forearms (Sitting or Standing)

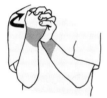

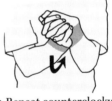

- Interlace fingers in front of you.
- Rotate hands and wrists clockwise 10 times.

- Repeat counterclockwise 10 times.

- Separate and straighten fingers until tension of stretch is felt.
- Hold 10 seconds.

- Relax, then bend fingers at knuckles and hold 10 seconds.
- Repeat first stretch once more.

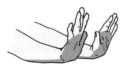

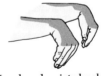

- With arms extended, palms down, bend wrists and raise fingertips.
- Hold 10 seconds.

- Now bend wrists back in opposite direction, fingers pointing down.
- Hold 10 seconds.

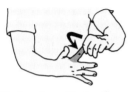

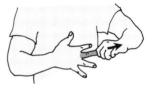

- With thumb and index finger, hold finger or thumb of opposite hand.
- Rotate 5 times clockwise, then 5 times counterclockwise.
- Rotate each finger and thumb.

- Next, gently pull finger straight out and hold 2–3 seconds.
- Do same thing with each finger and thumb.
- Repeat for your other hand.

- Now, shake arms and hands at sides for 10–12 seconds.
- Keep jaw relaxed and let shoulders hang downward as you shake out tension.

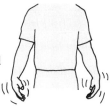

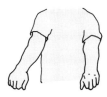
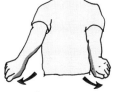

- Start with arms straight out in front.
- Slowly turn hands to outside until stretch is felt.
- Hold 5–10 seconds.

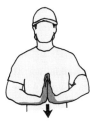

- Place hands palm-to-palm in front of you.
- Move hands downward, keeping palms together, until you feel a mild stretch.
- Keep elbows up and even.
- Hold 5–8 seconds.

- From above stretch, rotate palms around until they face more or less downward.
- Go until you feel a mild stretch.
- Keep elbows up and even.
- Hold 5–8 seconds.

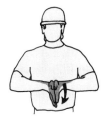

- Place hands palm-to-palm in front of you.
- Push one hand gently to side until you feel a mild stretch.
- Keep elbows up and even.
- Hold 5–8 seconds.

Use some or all of these stretches to counteract the problems that may come from repetitive movements, such as computer work. Use these daily, especially at work.

Sitting Stretches

A series of stretches you can do while sitting: These are good for people who work at office jobs. You can relieve tension and energize parts of your body that have become stiff from sitting.

Sitting stretches for upper body:

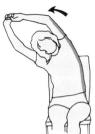

- Interlace fingers, then straighten arms out in front of you.
- Palms should be facing away from you.
- Feel stretch in arms and through upper part of back (shoulder blades).
- Hold stretch 10 seconds.

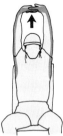

- Interlace fingers, then turn palms upward above head as you straighten arms.
- Think of elongating arms as you feel a stretch through arms and upper sides of rib cage.
- Hold 10 seconds.
- Excellent for slumping shoulders.
- Breathe deeply.

- With arms extended overhead, hold onto outside of left hand with right hand.
- Pull left arm to side.
- Keep arms as straight and comfortable as possible.
- Do other side.

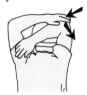

PNF Technique: *Contract — Relax — Stretch.*
- Hold right elbow with left hand.
- Move right elbow downward as you resist this movement with left hand (isometric contraction) for 3–4 seconds.

- After relaxing a moment, gently pull elbow over, behind head until you feel a mild stretch in back of upper arm.
- Hold 5–15 seconds.
- Repeat on other side.

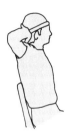
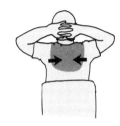

- Sit with fingers interlaced behind head, elbows straight out to sides, upper body aligned.
- Pull shoulder blades together to create feeling of tension through upper back and shoulder blades.
- Hold 5 seconds, relax.
- Repeat 1–3 times.

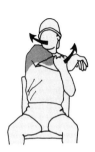

- Hold right arm just above elbow with left hand.
- As you look over right shoulder, gently pull elbow toward opposite shoulder until stretch is felt.
- Hold 10 seconds.
- Do both sides.

A Stretch for Forearms:

- With the palm of hand flat, thumb to outside and fingers pointed backward, slowly lean back to stretch forearm.
- Keep palms flat.
- Hold 10 seconds.
- Do both sides, or you can stretch both forearms at same time.

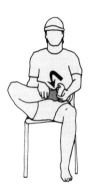

Sitting Stretches for Ankles, Side of Hip, and Lower Back

- While sitting, rotate ankles clockwise and then counterclockwise.
- Do one ankle at a time, 20–30 revolutions.

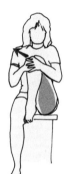

- Hold onto lower left leg just below knee.
- Gently pull it toward chest.
- Use left arm to pull bent leg across and toward opposite shoulder.
- Hold 15 seconds at easy stretch tension.
- Do both sides.

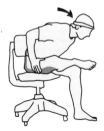

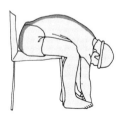

- Cross right leg over left leg, right ankle and foot resting just outside of left knee.
- Slowly lean upper body forward, bending from hips until you feel mild stretch.
- Hold 5–15 seconds.
- Repeat, crossing left leg over right leg.

- Lean forward to stretch.
- Keep head down, neck relaxed.
- Hold 10–20 seconds.
- Use hands to push yourself upright.

Stretches for the Face and Neck

This is a good stretch to use at the first signs of tightness or tension in the shoulder and neck area.

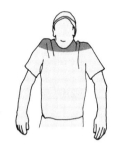

- Raise top of shoulders toward ears until you feel slight tension in neck and shoulders.
- Hold 3–5 seconds, then relax shoulders downward into normal position.
- Think: "Shoulders hang, shoulders down."

- Sit or stand with arms hanging loosely at sides.
- Turn head to one side, then to the other.
- Hold 5 seconds, each side.
- Keep shoulders relaxed and down.
- Do not hold breath.

This stretch may cause people around you to think you are a bit weird, but you often find a lot of tension in your face from frowning or squinting because of eye strain.

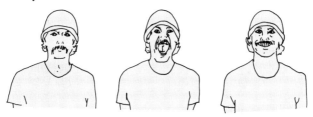

• Raise eyebrows and open eyes wide.
• At the same time, open mouth to stretch facial muscles.
• Hold 5 seconds.

Caution: If you hear clicking or popping noises when opening your mouth, check with your dentist.

SUMMARY OF SITTING STRETCHES

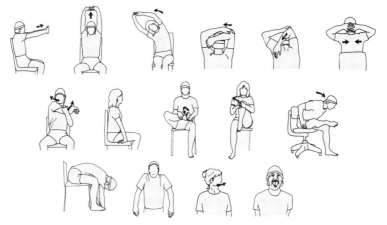

Do these sitting stretches, in this order, as a routine.

Advanced Stretches for the Legs and Groin with Feet Elevated

A wall or doorway can be useful for stretching the legs while you relax on your back. When doing these stretches think of the easy stretch, gradually increasing into the developmental stretch.

- Start with legs elevated and close together, butt about 3–5″ away from wall.
- Keep lower back flat and not arched or off floor.

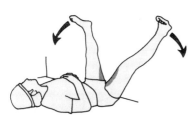

- Stretch groin from this position by slowly separating legs, with heels resting on wall, until you feel an easy stretch.
- Hold 30 seconds and relax.
- Breathe rhythmically.

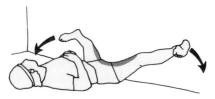

- As this position becomes easier over time, you can gradually stretch further by lowering legs.
- An advanced position is shown here. Do not try to copy this, but stretch within limits.
- Do not strain.
- The wall makes it possible to hold these stretches longer in a relaxed, stable position.

Remember to keep your butt 3–5 inches from the wall. If you are too close to the wall you may feel tightness in your lower back.

Variation:

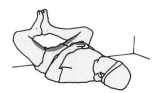

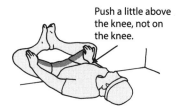

Push a little above the knee, not on the knee.

- Put soles of feet together, resting them against wall.
- Relax.

- To increase stretch, use hands to gently push down on inside of thighs.
- Relax while you stretch.
- Hold 10–15 seconds.

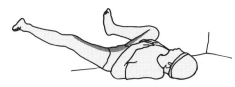

- To isolate and increase stretch in each side of groin area, straighten one leg out.
- Hold each leg 10–15 seconds.

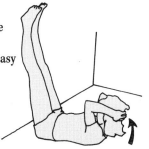

- To stretch neck from this position, interlace fingers behind head (at about ear level).
- Gently pull head forward until you feel an easy stretch.
- Hold 5 seconds.
- Repeat 2 or 3 times.

(See p. 27 for further information on neck stretches.)

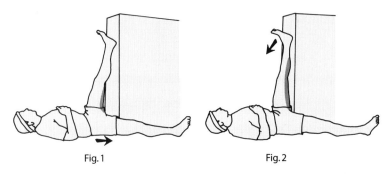

Fig. 1   Fig. 2

- An excellent way to stretch hamstrings:
- Lie on back with foot up on a doorway or wall and other leg in doorway or space where you can straighten it.
- Move body forward, toward doorway, until a mild stretch is felt *(fig. 1)*.
- Hold 10–15 seconds.
- To stretch calf and hamstrings from this position, bring toes toward shin until you feel a stretch in your calf *(fig. 2)*.
- Hold 10–15 seconds.

SUMMARY OF ADVANCED STRETCHES FOR THE LEGS AND GROIN WITH FEET ELEVATED

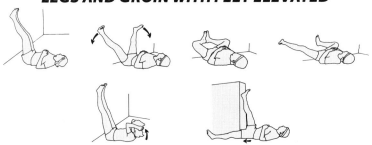

You can do these stretches, in this order, as a routine.

If you don't have much uninterrupted time available, use short periods of stretching (1–3 minutes) every three or four hours. This will help you to feel consistently good throughout the day.

Stretching the Groin and Hips with Legs Apart

The following stretches will make lateral movement easier, help maintain flexibility, and can prevent injuries. Gradually become accustomed to these stretches, which are primarily for the center of your body.

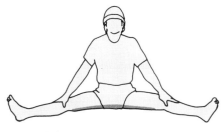 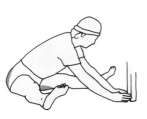

- Sit with feet a comfortable distance apart.
- Slowly lean forward from hips.
- Keep quadriceps relaxed and feet upright.
- Hold 10–20 seconds.
- Keep hands out in front for balance and stability or hold onto something for greater control.
- Breathe deeply.

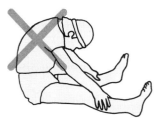

- Do not lean forward with head and shoulders.
- This will cause upper back to round and put pressure on lower back.
- If, when you lean forward, lower back is rounded (causing hips to tilt backward), it is because hips, lower back, and hamstrings are tight.
- To bend from hips correctly, you must keep lower back straight (upright) so you can move forward from hips and not by rounding back.

Don't stretch to be flexible. Stretch to feel good.

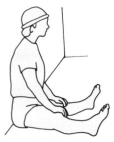

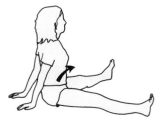

- A good way to adapt your hips and lower back gradually to a proper, upright position is to sit with lower back flat against wall.
- Hold easy stretch for 30 seconds.

- Another way is to sit with hands behind you.
- Using arms as a support will help lengthen spine as you concentrate on moving hips slightly forward.
- Hold 20 seconds.

Do not bend forward until you are able to feel comfortable doing the variations above. Get your body used to these positions before you try to stretch any further.

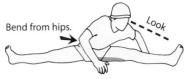

Bend from hips.   Look

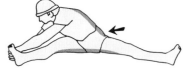

Variation:

- To stretch left hamstrings and right side of back, slowly bend forward from hips, toward foot of left leg.
- Keep chin in and back straight.
- Hold a good stretch 10–15 seconds.
- If necessary, use towel.
- Don't look down. Look just over toes.

Variation:

- Reach across body with left hand to right foot, putting right hand out to right side for balance. (This stretch requires good, overall flexibility.)
- This will increase stretch in hamstrings and in back, as far up as shoulder blades and as far down as hips.
- Do across-the-body stretch in both directions.
- Hold 5–15 seconds.

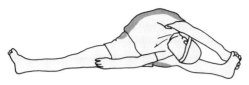

An Advanced Stretch:

- Reach overhead with hand and grasp opposite foot.
- Keep other arm resting close to body in front of you.
- Hold 5–15 seconds.
- Do both sides.

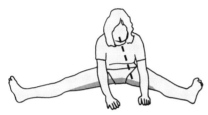

- Learn to hold stretch tensions at various angles.
- Stretch forward, left, and right, then teach yourself to hold stretches at angles toward left of center and right of center.
- Use same leg and upper body alignment as previously described.
- Hold 5–15 seconds. Stretch with complete self-control.

If you feel and look tight doing these stretches, do not be discouraged. Stretch without worrying about flexibility. Then you can gradually adapt your body to these new angles with stretch tensions that feel right.

A More Advanced Groin Stretch:

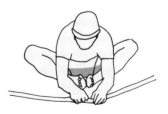

- Hold soles of feet together.
- Lean forward and hold onto something near floor in front of you (edge of mat, chair leg, etc.).
- Pull forward slowly to increase stretch.
- Do not overstretch.
- Hold and relax 10–20 seconds.
- Holding onto something will stabilize legs and make it easier to hold stretch when you are sitting with legs apart.

- Sitting on corner of mat, place legs and feet along outside edges.
- Find position where it is easy to relax while you feel slight stretch.
- Hold 10–15 seconds.
- Use hands behind you for balance and support.

Keep quads relaxed.

Keep toes and feet relaxed and upright.

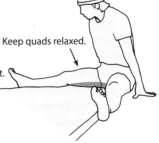

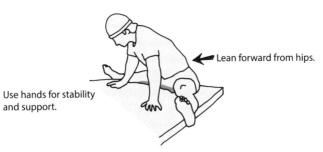

Lean forward from hips.

Use hands for stability and support.

- To increase stretch, move butt and hips forward.
- Slide legs down along the sides of mat.
- Toes and feet upright.

- Do not let legs turn in or out.
- Good stretch for limbering up groin and hips.

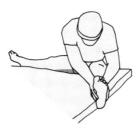

- To stretch one leg at a time, turn to face one foot and bend forward from hips in that direction.
- Reach down with hands and hold leg at point that gives you an easy stretch.
- Sit up and stretch other leg same way.
- Stretch tightest leg first. Relax.

- You can use towel around bottom of foot to help with this stretch.
- Hold easy stretch 5–15 seconds. No bouncing.
- Good stretch for hamstrings, lower back, and hips.

Learning the Splits

This section is for a limited number of people. Unless you are training for gymnastics, dance, or need extreme flexibility (as does an ice hockey goalkeeper, or a first baseman, or a ballet dancer), the other sections in this book should handle most of your stretching needs. I'm not trying to discourage you, but for everyday living being able to do the splits is hardly necessary!

> **Note:** Be sure to do an adequate warm-up prior to these stretches. Do some easier stretches and 5–6 minutes of aerobic activity.

Forward Splits

- From stretch position described on p. 51, slowly move front foot forward until you feel controlled stretch in back of legs and groin.
- Think of hips going straight down.
- Hold 10–15 seconds.

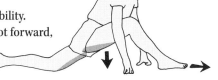

- Move front foot a little farther forward into developmental stretch.
- Hold 5–15 seconds.
- Use hands for balance and stability.
- The farther you move front foot forward, the more sole of foot will rise off floor.

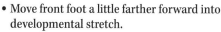

> A good way to prepare for the splits is to do the stretches on pp. 94–100.

- As you become more flexible, continue to move front foot forward as you lower hips.
- Keep shoulders directly above hips and back vertical.
- Hold 10–15 seconds.
- Repeat other side.

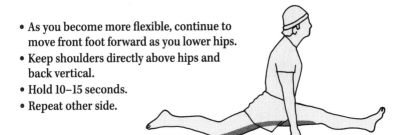

Learning to do the splits takes time and regular practice. Be sure not to overstretch. Let your body gradually adapt to the changes needed to accomplish the splits comfortably. Do not be in a rush and injure yourself.

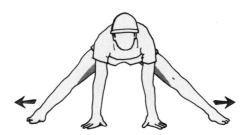

Side Splits
- Stand with feet pointed straight ahead.
- Gradually spread legs until you feel stretch on inside of upper legs.
- Think of hips going straight down.
- Use hands for balance.
- Hold easy stretch 5–15 seconds.

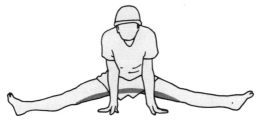

- As you become more limber, keep moving feet apart until desired stretch is created.
- As you get lower in this stretch, keep feet upright, with heels on floor.
- This will keep stretch on inside of upper legs and extreme tension off ligaments of knees. (If you keep feet flat on floor there is a possibility of overstretching inside ligament of knees.)
- Hold 5–15 seconds.
- As body gradually adapts, slowly increase stretch by lowering hips a bit further.
- *Be careful of overstretching.*

Doing the stretches below will help you in learning the splits.

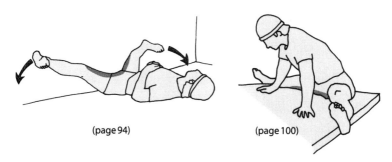

(page 94)   (page 100)

STRETCHING
ROUTINES
Everyday Activities

These are stretching routines that can help you in dealing with the muscular tension and tightness of everyday life. There are routines for different age groups, different body parts, different occupations and activities, as well as stretches to do spontaneously at odd moments throughout the day. Once you learn how to stretch, you will be able to develop your own routines to suit your own particular needs.

When you first do the routines, you can look up the instructions for each stretch in the page numbers listed. After a while you will know how to stretch without looking at the instructions each time.

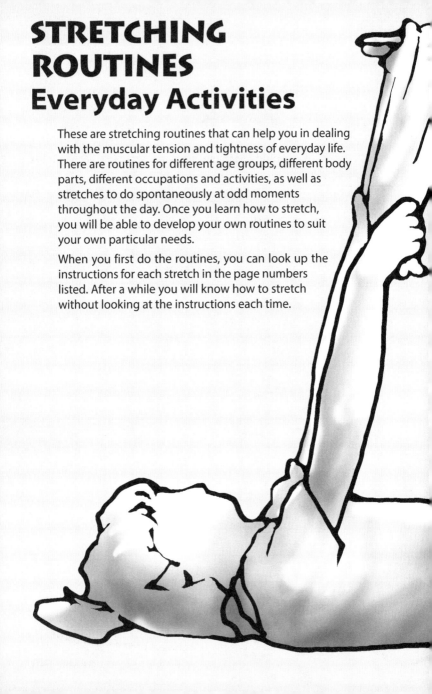

IN THE MORNING

Start the day with some relaxed stretches so your body can function more naturally. Tight and stiff muscles will feel good from comfortable stretching. The first four stretches can be done in bed before you get up. After arising and you've moved around a bit, do the next four stretches.

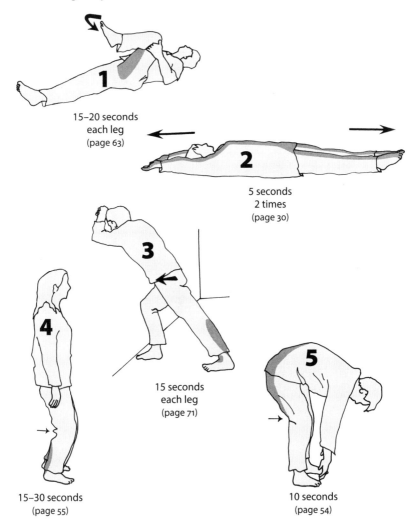

1 15–20 seconds
each leg
(page 63)

2 5 seconds
2 times
(page 30)

3 15 seconds
each leg
(page 71)

4 15–30 seconds
(page 55)

5 10 seconds
(page 54)

Stretching: Pocket Book Edition © 2021 by Bob and Jean Anderson. Shelter Publications, Inc.

APPROXIMATELY 2 MINUTES

This is a great time to stretch every day. These stretches will relax your body and help you to sleep more soundly. Take your time, and *feel* the body parts being stretched. Stretch lightly, breathe deeply, and be relaxed.

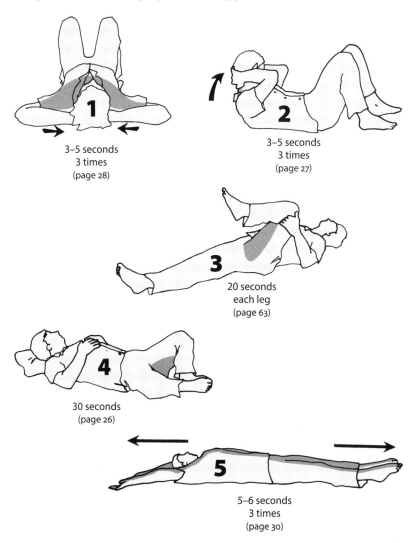

1

3–5 seconds
3 times
(page 28)

2

3–5 seconds
3 times
(page 27)

3

20 seconds
each leg
(page 63)

4

30 seconds
(page 26)

5

5–6 seconds
3 times
(page 30)

EVERYDAY STRETCHES

APPROXIMATELY 5 MINUTES

Start with several minutes of walking. Then use these everyday stretches to fine-tune your muscles. This is a general routine that emphasizes stretching and relaxing the muscles most frequently used during normal day-to-day activities.

In the simple tasks of everyday living, we often use our body in strained or awkward ways, creating stress and tension. A kind of muscular *rigor mortis* sets in. If you can set aside 10 minutes every day for stretching, you will offset this accumulated tension so you can use your body with greater ease.

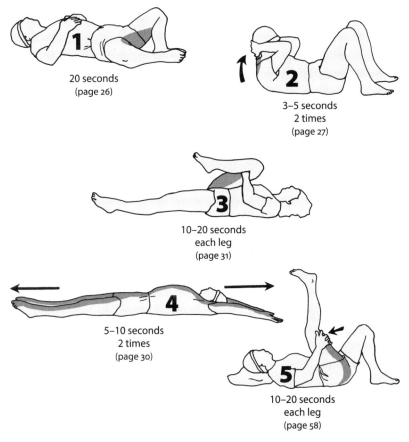

1
20 seconds
(page 26)

2
3–5 seconds
2 times
(page 27)

3
10–20 seconds
each leg
(page 31)

4
5–10 seconds
2 times
(page 30)

5
10–20 seconds
each leg
(page 58)

     Stretching: Pocket Book Edition © 2021 by Bob and Jean Anderson. Shelter Publications, Inc.

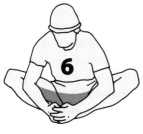

20–30 seconds
(page 58)

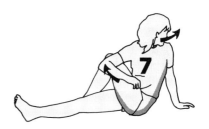

8–10 seconds
each side
(page 60)

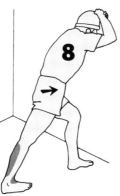

10–15 seconds
each leg
(page 71)

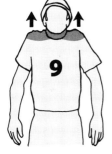

4–5 seconds
2 times
(page 46)

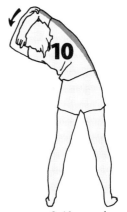

8–10 seconds
each side
(page 44)

APPROXIMATELY 4 MINUTES

This series of stretches works for repetitive stress problems in the hands and arms. Breathe naturally, stay comfortable, and be relaxed as you stretch.

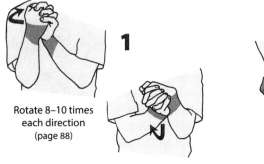
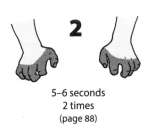

Rotate 8–10 times
each direction
(page 88)

5–6 seconds
2 times
(page 88)

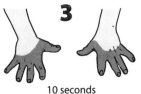

10 seconds
2 times
(page 88)

10 seconds
each position
(page 88)

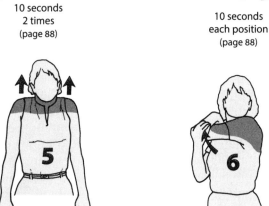

3–5 seconds
3 times
(page 46)

15 seconds
each arm
(page 43)

Stretching: Pocket Book Edition © 2021 by Bob and Jean Anderson. Shelter Publications, Inc.

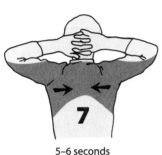

7

5–6 seconds
2 times
(page 28)

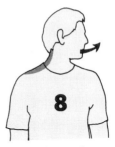

8

5–10 seconds
each side
(page 92)

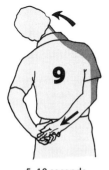

9

5–10 seconds
each arm
(page 47)

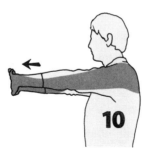

10

20 seconds
(page 45)

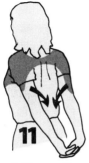

11

5–10 seconds
(page 47)

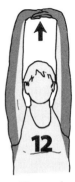

12

15 seconds
(page 46)

APPROXIMATELY 5 MINUTES

Many people carry stress in their neck and shoulder area. This stretching routine will help with that problem. Do these stretches throughout the day. Breathe deeply and relax.

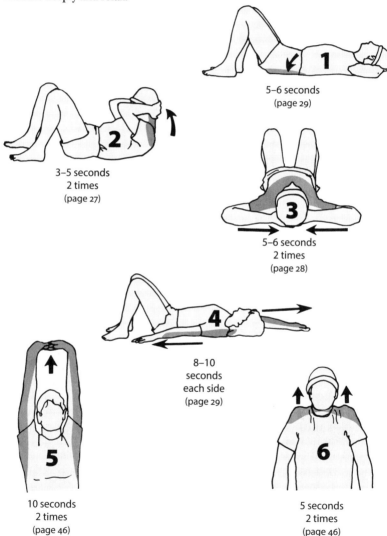

1
5–6 seconds
(page 29)

2
3–5 seconds
2 times
(page 27)

3
5–6 seconds
2 times
(page 28)

4
8–10
seconds
each side
(page 29)

5
10 seconds
2 times
(page 46)

6
5 seconds
2 times
(page 46)

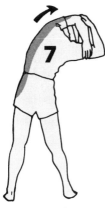

7

8–10 seconds
each side
(page 44)

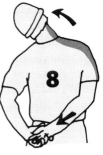

8

8–10 seconds
each side
2 times
(page 44)

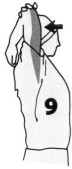

9

5–15 seconds
each arm
2 times
(page 44)

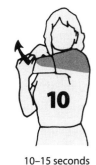

10

10–15 seconds
each arm
(page 43)

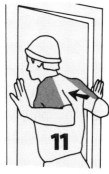

11

15–20 seconds
(page 47)

12

15–20 seconds
(page 81)

APPROXIMATELY 6 MINUTES

These stretches are designed for the relief of muscular low back pain and are also good for relieving tension in the upper back, shoulders, and neck. For best results do them every night just before going to sleep. Hold only stretch tensions that feel good to you. *Do not overstretch.*

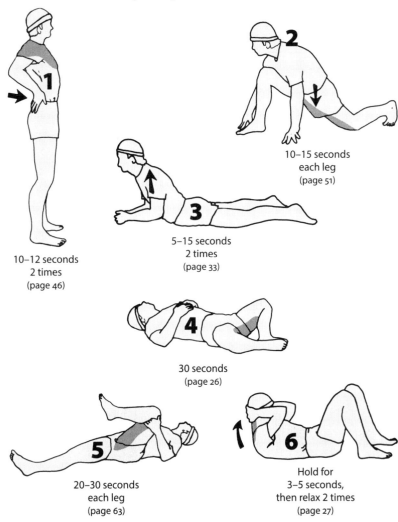

10–12 seconds
2 times
(page 46)

10–15 seconds
each leg
(page 51)

5–15 seconds
2 times
(page 33)

30 seconds
(page 26)

20–30 seconds
each leg
(page 63)

Hold for
3–5 seconds,
then relax 2 times
(page 27)

   Stretching: Pocket Book Edition © 2021 by Bob and Jean Anderson. Shelter Publications, Inc.

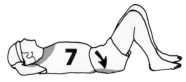

Contract
5–8 seconds,
then relax 2 times
(page 29)

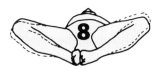

Rock gently
back and forth
15–20 times
(page 26)

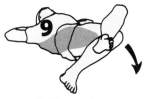

10–30 seconds
each leg
(page 27)

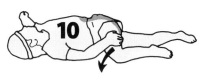

10–15 seconds
each leg
(page 32)

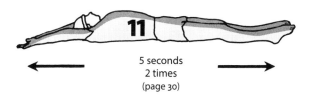

5 seconds
2 times
(page 30)

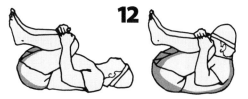

10–15 seconds
2 times
(page 63)

APPROXIMATELY 7 MINUTES

Stretch comfortably after a light warm-up of walking in place or riding a stationary bike for 2–3 minutes. Remember to stretch with control as you gradually limber up. Relax and breathe rhythmically.

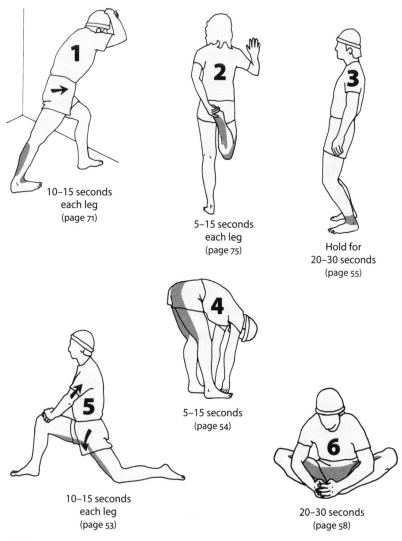

1 10–15 seconds
each leg
(page 71)

2 5–15 seconds
each leg
(page 75)

3 Hold for
20–30 seconds
(page 55)

4 5–15 seconds
(page 54)

5 10–15 seconds
each leg
(page 53)

6 20–30 seconds
(page 58)

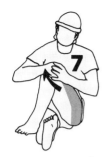

10–15 seconds
each leg
(page 61)

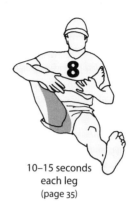

10–15 seconds
each leg
(page 35)

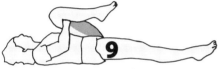

30 seconds
each leg
(page 31)

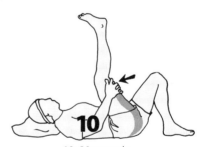

10–20 seconds
each leg
(page 58)

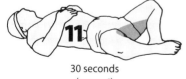

30 seconds
(page 26)

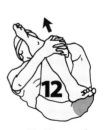

10–15 seconds
each leg
(page 36)

SPONTANEOUS STRETCHES

You can stretch at odd times of the day. Reading a paper, talking on the phone, waiting for a bus . . . these are times for easy, relaxed stretching. Be creative; think of stretches to do during normally wasted time.

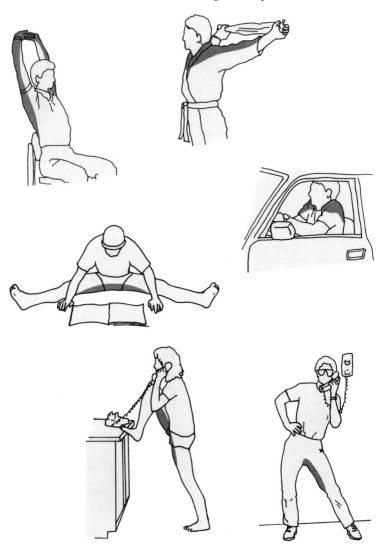

Stretching: Pocket Book Edition © 2021 by Bob and Jean Anderson. Shelter Publications, Inc.

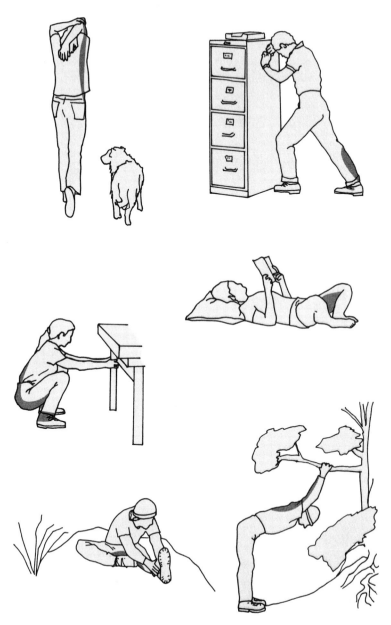

BLUE-COLLAR STRETCHES

APPROXIMATELY 5 MINUTES

Before you do any physical work — especially lifting — do some stretches. Stretching gives your muscles a signal they are about to be used, and a few minutes of stretching before starting work will make you feel better and help avoid injuries.

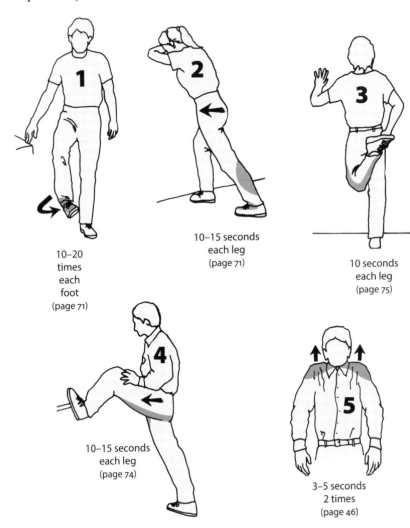

1
10–20 times each foot
(page 71)

2
10–15 seconds each leg
(page 71)

3
10 seconds each leg
(page 75)

4
10–15 seconds each leg
(page 74)

5
3–5 seconds 2 times
(page 46)

Stretching: Pocket Book Edition © 2021 by Bob and Jean Anderson. Shelter Publications, Inc.

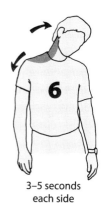

3–5 seconds
each side
(page 46)

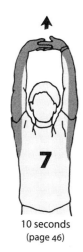

10 seconds
(page 46)

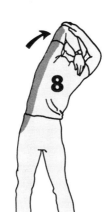

8–10 seconds
each side
(page 44)

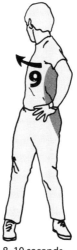

8–10 seconds
each side
(page 81)

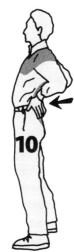

8–10 seconds
2 times
(page 46)

APPROXIMATELY 4 MINUTES

This is a series of stretches to do after sitting for a long time. The sitting position causes the blood to pool in the lower legs and feet, the hamstring muscles to tighten up, and the back and neck muscles to become stiff and tight. These stretches will improve your circulation and loosen up those areas that are tense from a prolonged period of sitting.

1

Walk a bit
for 2–3
minutes

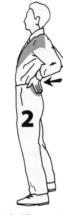

2

10–15 seconds
2 times
(page 46)

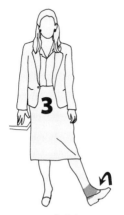

3

Rotate
each ankle
10–15
times
(page 71)

4

10 seconds
(page 46)

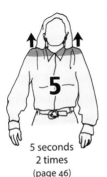

5

5 seconds
2 times
(page 46)

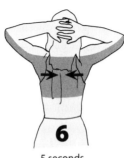

6

5 seconds
2 times
(page 28)

Stretching: Pocket Book Edition © 2021 by Bob and Jean Anderson. Shelter Publications, Inc.

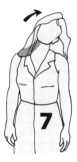

7

3–5 seconds
each side
(page 46)

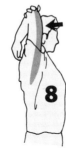

8

10 seconds
each arm
(page 44)

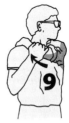

9

15 seconds
each arm
(page 43)

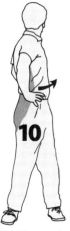

10

10–12 seconds
each side
(page 81)

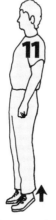

11

3–4 seconds
(page 71)

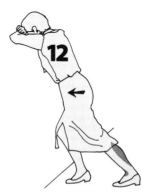

12

10–15 seconds
each leg
(page 71)

APPROXIMATELY 4 MINUTES

Before you do any work in the garden, do a few minutes of easy stretching. This will help get your body ready to work efficiently without the usual tightness and stiffness that results from this kind of work. Stretch to reduce muscle tension and make work easier.

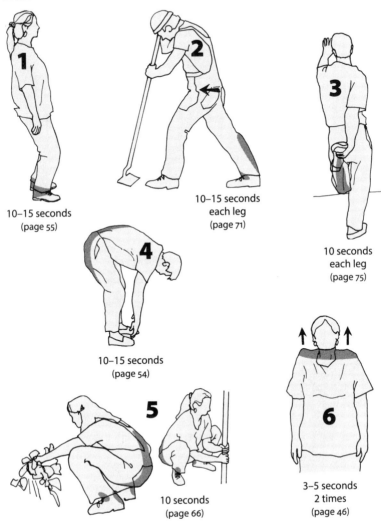

1 10–15 seconds
(page 55)

2 10–15 seconds
each leg
(page 71)

3 10 seconds
each leg
(page 75)

4 10–15 seconds
(page 54)

5 10 seconds
(page 66)

6 3–5 seconds
2 times
(page 46)

Stretching: Pocket Book Edition © 2021 by Bob and Jean Anderson. Shelter Publications, Inc.

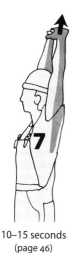

7

10–15 seconds
(page 46)

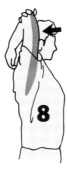

8

10 seconds
each arm
(page 44)

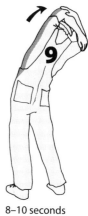

9

8–10 seconds
each side
(page 44)

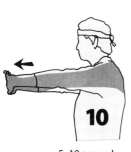

10

5–10 seconds
(page 45)

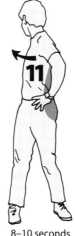

11

8–10 seconds
each side
(page 81)

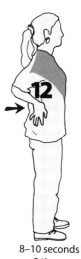

12

8–10 seconds
2 times
(page 46)

APPROXIMATELY 5 MINUTES

It is never too late to start stretching. In fact, the older we get, the more important it becomes to stretch on a regular basis.

With age and inactivity, the body gradually loses its range of motion; muscles can lose their elasticity and become weak and tight. But the body has an amazing capacity for the recovery of lost flexibility and strength if a regular program of fitness is followed.

The basic method of stretching is the same regardless of differences in age and flexibility. *Stretching properly means that you do not go beyond your comfortable limits.* You don't have to try to copy the drawings in this book. Learn to stretch your body without pushing too far; stretch by how you feel. It will take time to loosen up tight muscle groups that have been that way for years, but it can be done with patience and regularity. If you have any doubts about what you should be doing, consult your physician *before you start.*

Here is a series of stretches to help restore and maintain flexibility.

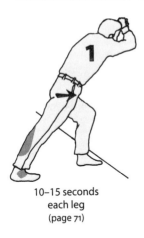

10–15 seconds
each leg
(page 71)

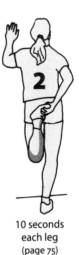

10 seconds
each leg
(page 75)

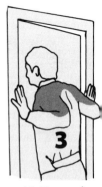

15–20 seconds
(page 47)

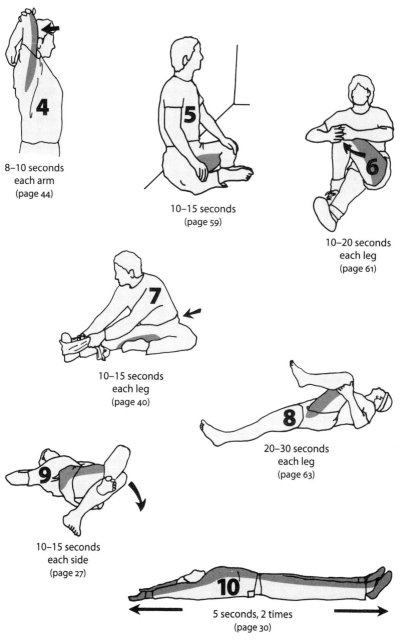

8–10 seconds
each arm
(page 44)

10–15 seconds
(page 59)

10–20 seconds
each leg
(page 61)

10–15 seconds
each leg
(page 40)

20–30 seconds
each leg
(page 63)

10–15 seconds
each side
(page 27)

5 seconds, 2 times
(page 30)

APPROXIMATELY 4 MINUTES

It's never too early to start stretching! Show your kids how to do these stretches (or show these to your kids' teachers, so they can get the whole class stretching). Explain to them that stretching is not a contest, and that they should stretch slowly, concentrating on the areas being stretched.

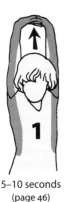

5–10 seconds
(page 46)

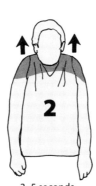

3–5 seconds
2 times
(page 46)

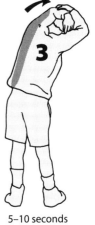

5–10 seconds
each side
(page 44)

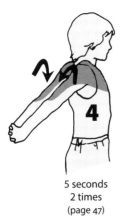

5 seconds
2 times
(page 47)

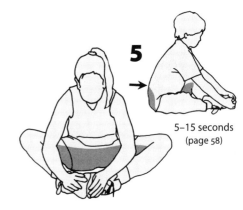

5–15 seconds
(page 58)

Stretching: Pocket Book Edition © 2021 by Bob and Jean Anderson. Shelter Publications, Inc.

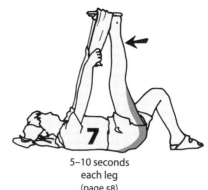

5–10 seconds
each leg
(page 58)

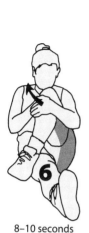

8–10 seconds
each leg
(page 61)

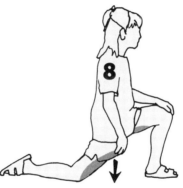

10 seconds
each leg
(page 51)

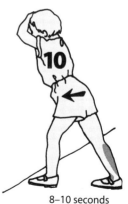

8–10 seconds
each leg
(page 71)

5–10 seconds
each leg
(page 75)

Many people think they don't have enough time to stretch, yet watch several hours of television a night. Well, you can stretch as you watch TV. This will not interfere with your viewing and you will be accomplishing something during otherwise sedentary times.

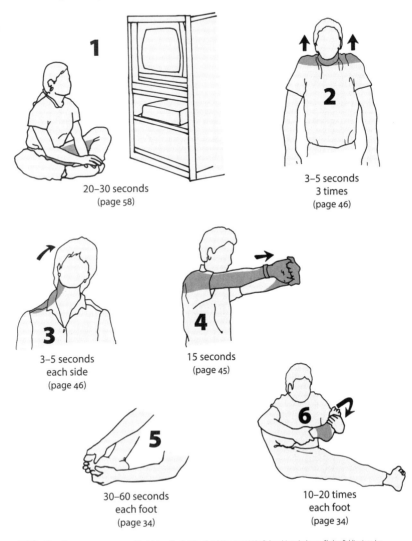

1
20–30 seconds
(page 58)

2
3–5 seconds
3 times
(page 46)

3
3–5 seconds
each side
(page 46)

4
15 seconds
(page 45)

5
30–60 seconds
each foot
(page 34)

6
10–20 times
each foot
(page 34)

Stretching: Pocket Book Edition © 2021 by Bob and Jean Anderson. Shelter Publications, Inc.

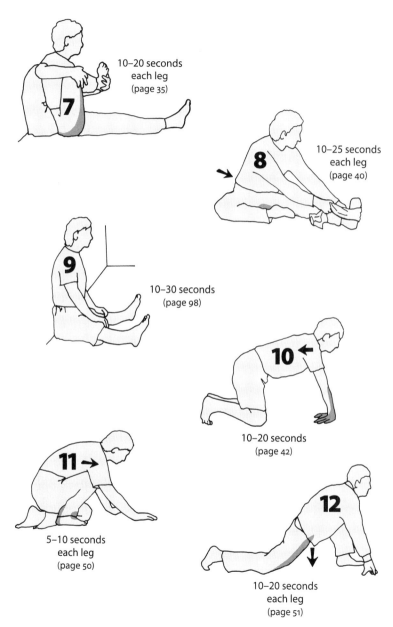

10–20 seconds
each leg
(page 35)

10–25 seconds
each leg
(page 40)

10–30 seconds
(page 98)

10–20 seconds
(page 42)

5–10 seconds
each leg
(page 50)

10–20 seconds
each leg
(page 51)

APPROXIMATELY 5 MINUTES

These stretches will make the movements of walking feel free and easy.
Warm up by walking several minutes before stretching.

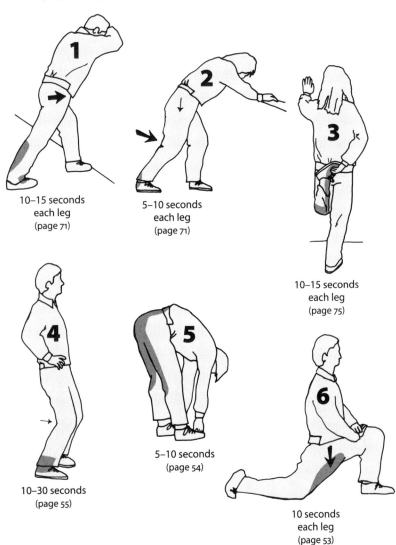

10–15 seconds
each leg
(page 71)

5–10 seconds
each leg
(page 71)

10–15 seconds
each leg
(page 75)

10–30 seconds
(page 55)

5–10 seconds
(page 54)

10 seconds
each leg
(page 53)

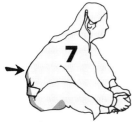

7

10–15 seconds
(page 58)

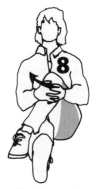

8

5–10 seconds
each side
(page 61)

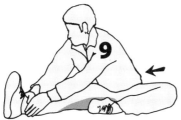

9

10–15 seconds
each leg
(page 39)

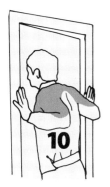

10

10–20 seconds
(page 47)

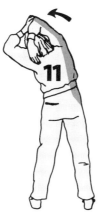

11

8–10 seconds
each side
(page 44)

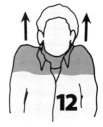

12

5 seconds
2 times
(page 46)

TRAVELERS' STRETCHES

APPROXIMATELY 2 MINUTES

Stretch at various times throughout your journey to help your body
feel less stiff and tight.

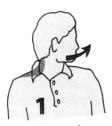

1

3–5 seconds
each side
(page 92)

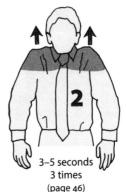

2

3–5 seconds
3 times
(page 46)

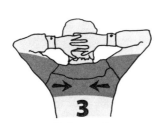

3

3–5 seconds
(page 91)

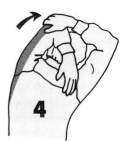

4

5 seconds
each side
(page 44)

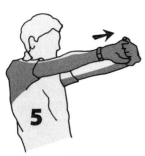

5

15 seconds
(page 90)

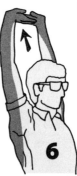

6

8–10 seconds
(page 90)

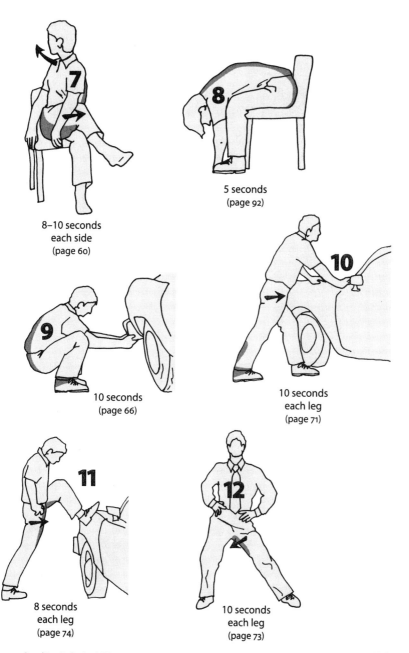

7

8–10 seconds
each side
(page 60)

8

5 seconds
(page 92)

9

10 seconds
(page 66)

10

10 seconds
each leg
(page 71)

11

8 seconds
each leg
(page 74)

12

10 seconds
each leg
(page 73)

AIRPLANE STRETCHES

Photocopy these pages and take them along on your next flight. Stretching on the plane will relieve stress and stiffness and allow you to arrive in a more relaxed state. Don't be surprised if your fellow passengers follow your example and start stretching too. Especially good to do just before you land.

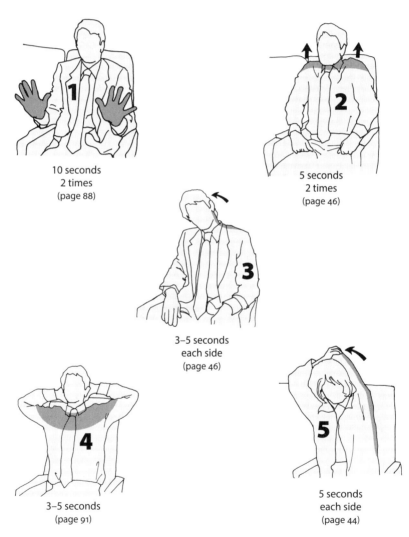

10 seconds
2 times
(page 88)

5 seconds
2 times
(page 46)

3–5 seconds
each side
(page 46)

3–5 seconds
(page 91)

5 seconds
each side
(page 44)

Stretching: Pocket Book Edition © 2021 by Bob and Jean Anderson. Shelter Publications, Inc.

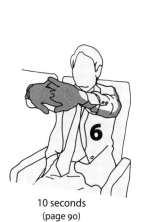

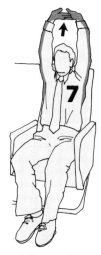

10 seconds
(page 90)

8–10 seconds
(page 90)

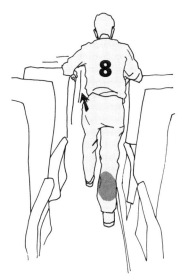

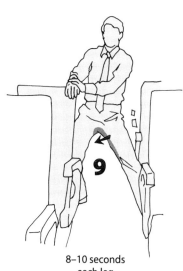

10–12 seconds
each leg
(page 71)

8–10 seconds
each leg
(page 73)

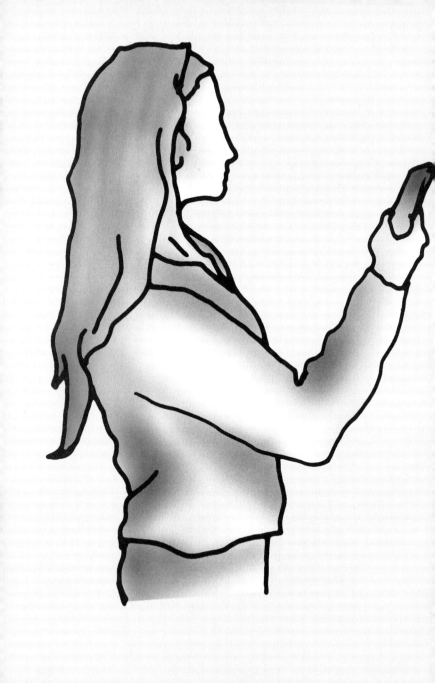

STRETCHING IN THE AGE OF COMPUTERS AND SMARTPHONES

Computers

Ten years ago, we updated this book to address the problems coming from sedentary office work, especially from too much time spent at a computer.

People were staying in the same position for long periods of time while working on computers. Even typewriters that were in usage earlier required some movement: putting in paper, turning the roller knob, working the carriage release lever. Computers eliminated these functions.

Phones
What's new?

The last ten years have seen a tremendous increase in smartphone usage, and this has caused problems, especially poor posture from looking downward most of the time.

In this section of the book, we'll outline the main problems that come from spending a lot of time on a computer and/or phone each day, and present simple stretches and tips that will improve your posture, make you feel better, and minimize pain.

Desk (Computer) Fitness

Sitting for hours at a time is a relatively recent phenomenon in human history. These days, most people working on computers sit for too long without a break, and problems are multiplying.

Computer Injuries

Fast, light-touch keyboards that allow high-speed typing have resulted in an epidemic of injuries to the hands, arms, and shoulders. Slowly, the thousands of repeated keystrokes and long periods of gripping and dragging a mouse damage the body. This happens even more quickly due to improper keyboarding technique and/or body positions that stress the tendons and nerves in the hand, wrist, arms, shoulders, and neck.

Typical problems

- **Repetitive strain injuries** — RSIs — (such as carpal tunnel syndrome and tendinitis) are typically caused by repetitive hand movements.
- **Back pain:** Sitting for long periods compresses your spine. If your posture is bad, gravity accentuates the problem.
- **Stiff muscles:** Not moving for long periods can cause neck and shoulder pain.
- **Tight joints:** Inactivity can cause joints to tighten, which makes moving more difficult or even painful.
- **Poor circulation:** When you sit very still, blood settles in the lower legs and feet and does not circulate well. There can be tingling, coldness, or numbness in the hands, and back pain.

What If You Have Such Symptoms?

We all have occasional aches and pains that go away in a day or two. But if you have recurring problems from using the computer, run, do not walk, to your doctor or health care provider. An early diagnosis can limit damage. Don't ignore the pain; you may sustain a serious injury. There are no quick fixes. No wrist splint, arm rest, split keyboard, spinal adjustment, etc. is going to get you right back to work at full speed. Even carpal tunnel sufferers who have wrist release surgery can be back in pain if they don't make long-term changes in their techniques and work habits. Healing does happen but it may take months, not days.

Ergonomics Modern-day office ergonomics is the science of providing furniture, tools, and equipment that improve the comfort, safety, and health of office workers. Some basic principles:

- **Keyboard** should be set at a height so that forearms, wrists, and hands are aligned when keyboarding, and parallel to the floor, or bent slightly down from elbow to hand — the hands are never bent back.

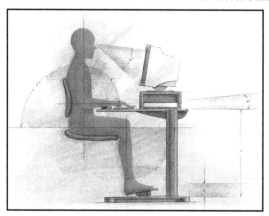

  Preferably the stand or desk on which the keyboard sits is adjustable. There are many ergonomic keyboards available, some of them quite unusual.

- **Mouse pad** should be at a height where your arm, wrist, and hand are aligned and in "neutral." It's good if the stand or desk the mouse pad sits on is also adjustable.

- **Wrists**, while you are actually typing, should not rest on anything, and should not be bent up, down, or to the side, but should be in a straight line with your forearm, as viewed from above. Your arms should move your hands around, and instead of resting your wrists, stretch to hit keys with your fingers.

- **Chair** should be adjustable and comfortable. Set it so that your thighs are either parallel to the floor or at a slight downward angle from the hips to the knees. Sit straight, not slouching, and not straining forward to reach the keys. Stay relaxed.

Further Tips

- **Sit *and* stand.** Movement is important. Try adjusting the height or angle of your chair after a few hours, or stand after sitting for a period. In fact, the least stressful working position is one where the individual can "sit *and* stand" rather than "sit *or* stand." Many people now use standup mats or "anti-fatigue mats" that provide support and cushioning while standing.

- **Don't pound the keys.** Use a light touch.

- **Use two hands** to perform double-key operations such as **Command-P**, **Ctrl-C** or **Alt-F**, instead of twisting one hand to do them.

- **Hold the mouse lightly.** Don't grip it hard or squeeze it. Place it where you don't have to reach up or over very far to use it (close to the keyboard is best).

- **Use the tap-to-click setting for your trackpad.** Then you don't have to hold your thumb down to click or drag, and it puts less strain on your thumb and wrist.

- **Keep your arms and hands warm.** Cold muscles and tendons are at much greater risk for overuse injuries, and many offices are overly air-conditioned. Fingerless gloves help a lot.

- **Rest.** When you stop typing for a while, rest your hands in your lap and/or on their sides instead of leaving them on the keyboard.

- **Stretch.** Stretch frequently throughout the day. *(See pages 132–135.)*

- **Elevate your feet.** Elevating your feet daily for 5–10 minutes can help circulation. A very healthy habit.

- **Move.** Get up and move whenever you can. If possible, walk to talk to a near-by colleague instead of using the phone. Try using the stairs (at least for some floors) instead of the elevator.

- **Take breaks.** Some experts suggest a 10-second break every 3 minutes, others suggest a 1-minute break every 15 minutes, a 5-minute break every half hour, or a 15-minute break every 2 hours, etc. You can stretch and/or move around during these breaks.

- **Use a TheraCane®.** This is an excellent body tool to work out upper body tightness and tension. *(See page 235.)*

- **Breathing** Deep diaphragmatic breathing every hour helps you to reduce stress, create calmness and mental focus. If you are not sure you are using your diaphragm when breathing. (*See page 227*, the Breath Builder, a tool to improve your diaphragmatic breath.)

What Can Stretching Do?

- If you aren't injured, use the stretches on pages 132–135. Stretch regularly a few times a day and it may help you minimize repetitive strain injuries.
- If you are injured, take this book to your doctor or health care provider and ask which of the stretching programs you can follow. Point out that the stretching prescriptions on pages 228–229 can be used to customize a series of stretches for your particular condition.
- On the following four pages are stretching programs specifically designed for people who work at computers.

Healing Takes Time

If you have a repetitive strain injury, don't expect an instant cure. Many people have found that after a few months of following good ergonomic principles and stretching regularly, their condition has improved.

APPROXIMATELY 1¼ MINUTES

Many people do not understand this, but working on a keyboard all day, day after day, is physically demanding. Repetitive strain injuries (RSIs) from mouse and keyboard use have risen dramatically. The routine below is designed for keyboard operators and their potential (or actual) problems.

- If you are injured, see a doctor (preferably one with RSI experience) for advice on which stretches will help you recover.
- If you are not injured now, do these stretches throughout the day as preventive medicine. (Stretch while making "saves," for example.)
- *See pp. 140–145, for more on RSI problems.*

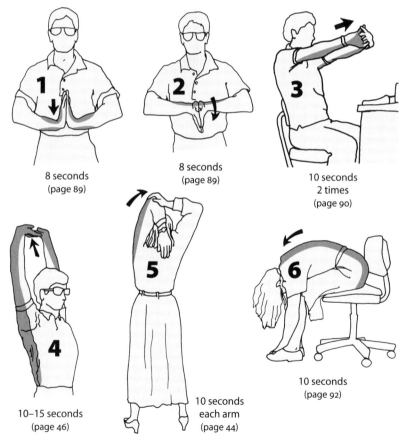

8 seconds
(page 89)

8 seconds
(page 89)

10 seconds
2 times
(page 90)

10–15 seconds
(page 46)

10 seconds
each arm
(page 44)

10 seconds
(page 92)

APPROXIMATELY 1 MINUTE

No matter how fast your modem, you're always waiting for something to load while online. (This will probably never change, for even as modems get faster and faster, files get larger and larger.) These stretches are for your upper body, especially neck, shoulders, and wrists.

- Whenever you are reading online, and not using the keyboard or mouse, you can do upper body stretches using both arms.
- After you follow this program a few times, you'll know these stretches by heart; thereafter do them frequently while online.

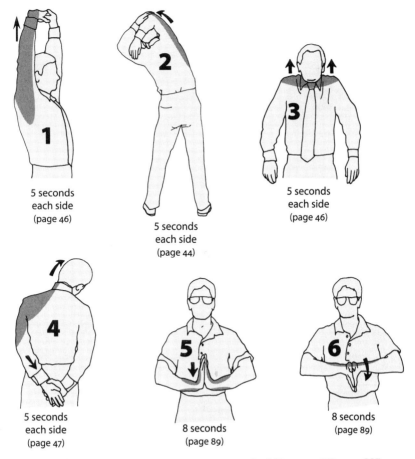

1
5 seconds
each side
(page 46)

2
5 seconds
each side
(page 44)

3
5 seconds
each side
(page 46)

4
5 seconds
each side
(page 47)

5
8 seconds
(page 89)

6
8 seconds
(page 89)

Phone Health Problems

Google research indicates there were between 3–4 billion smartphone users worldwide in 2019, and that number is growing.

According to RescueTime, an app for iOS and Android phones, people in 2019 spent an average of 3–4 hours every day on their smartphones, with 20% of users spending 4½ hours.

It sneaked up on us. Smartphones are life-changing devices, so useful and compelling that we've overlooked a major downside: bad posture! Which leads to back problems, among other things.

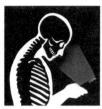 If you look at teenagers, they're invariably looking at their phones, heads bent forward, posture off-balance. Young people get off to a bad start in life when they unwittingly develop bad posture from bending over and staring at a small screen for hours on end. Unwittingly, because it's a gradual process, like the frog placed in a pot of slowly warming water.

The same goes for adults. The next time you're in the streets, or are in a market, or on public transit, notice how people are bent over, looking at their phones.

(This isn't due entirely to phones: we hunch over when reading, driving, even walking. The head is almost always out of balance.)

The repetitive use of fingers (or thumbs) can contribute to repetitive stress injuries such as tendinitis or carpal tunnel syndrome.

Symptoms of tech neck (or text neck) are not just a stiff neck, but pain between shoulder blades, and sometimes headaches. Worse, over time, tendons and joints can become damaged and slouching permanent.

Poor posture while sitting, standing, walking, or looking at your phone can lead to more than upper body pain and stiffness; poor posture affects other parts of the spine, such as the middle and low back. Once sustained, these types of injuries are difficult to treat. Tendons are not muscles that tighten and contract, so tendon damage is hard to repair.

We encourage you to do some web research on the subject. Start by googling "tech neck"; there's a ton of information out there. We also encourage you to seek advice from a health care professional if you are having problems.

Tech Neck

Tech neck is a phrase describing neck (and shoulder) soreness that results from tucking your head down over your chin (sometimes called "hunchback slouch") while looking down at a phone screen. This causes the muscles in the back of your neck to contract in order to hold the head up.

An adult head weighs 10 to 11 pounds. As the angle of leaning forward increases, there's increasing stress on your spine. A 15-degree forward tilt is said to put a strain on your neck of 27 pounds (10 pounds from weight of the head, 17 pounds from imbalance).

Looking down at smart phones for long periods of time can cause the bones in the neck to mold into a curved position.

Text Neck

Text neck refers to the problems that come from *texting* on a phone.

The dangers of texting while driving are obvious, but there's also danger in texting while walking; there's been an increase in pedestrian accidents from people texting while walking. Some cities have even considered making texting while walking illegal.

Texting requires more concentration than talking and/or using voice recognition. (You can talk on a phone without staring at it.)

Posture Check – Standing

How's your posture right now? Are you standing balanced evenly on both feet, or are you standing predominantly on one foot? Is your head forward, causing rounded shoulders and tension in your neck, shoulders, and upper and lower back? How about your jaw? Is it being held tight because you are clenching your teeth, creating tension throughout your upper body? Are your hands relaxed, or are they being held tight, in an uncomfortable position?

Here are some ideas to help you get back in balance and reduce unwanted muscle tension and tightness:

• **Focus on your legs and feet.** Try standing with your feet pointed straight ahead, almost shoulder-width apart. Now make sure your legs are straight, but knees not locked backwards. Make sure you're standing evenly on both feet with your weight equally distributed between your two feet. This helps keep your center of gravity directed downward.

This is more of a position of power and relaxation than the position of weakness and instability that goes with standing with your weight on mostly one foot.

- **Next focus on your upper body and head.** While standing in a more balanced stance, lift your chest slightly upward while your head is lifted back above your shoulders. Your chin should be level to the floor/ground and you should be looking forward, not downward. Think: "Stand tall." Check your jaw to be sure it's relaxed. If not, simply say this to yourself: "Jaw relax," and unclench your teeth, letting your jaw relax slightly.
- *Focus on your shoulders.* Next, bring the top of your shoulders up toward your ears. Hold for 1–3 seconds. Repeat 3–5 times. Inhale as you bring your shoulders up; exhale as you bring them down. Say to yourself: "Shoulders hang, shoulders down."
- *Hands* If they are tight and tense, let them relax. Shake them out as on page 89. Think: "Hands relax."
- *Breathe* Learn to take at least 10 full diaphragmatic breaths every hour to help reduce stress.
- *Practice realigning yourself throughout the day.* This can reduce the pain and discomfort of poor posture.

During the day, do quick posture checks. If your shoulders are tight and tense, do some shoulder shrugs. If your jaw is relaxed, it will reduce the tension and tightness in your face and upper body. If you are standing out of balance, realign your legs and feet so that your weight is evenly distributed.

Three important things to practice:

1. Bring your phone up to eye level, rather than looking down.

2. Look down with your eyes, not your head.

3. Take a three-minute break for every 15 to 20 minutes you talk on the phone.

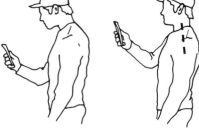

Your head controls your body.

Reducing Phone Stress

Google reports that "…mobile devices loaded with social media, email and news apps" are creating "…a constant sense of obligation, generating unintended personal stress." What can you do?

Turn off all notifications except for the ones you want to receive.

Delete apps or websites if they cause anxiety or stress. (Apps/websites like YouTube, Facebook, Twitter, WhatsApp, WeChat, TikTok, Instagram, etc. lure people into lots of time spent.)

Take breaks. Try a 24-hour "digital Sabbath." Many people who do this find an unexpected sense of peacefulness and calm without the digital leash and return to their devices refreshed.

There are books on how to "break up with your phone," that show you how to "…break up, then make up." The idea isn't to give up your phone, but to get a handle on usage, on hours spent.

Stretch! See *Phone Stretches* on the next two pages.

Phone Stickers

Here is an analog tool for your phone. It's not an app. It's a little printed reminder you can photo-copy and tape on the back of your phone. There are two versions, for different size phones. (Packing or shipping tape works very well here.)

If you want to stretch, no need to start up an app. Just turn your phone over and do a few stretches.

It also reminds you to hold your phone at eye level.

Photocopy this and tape to the back of your phone.
OR
Go to *shltr.net/phone-sticker* to download a color version.

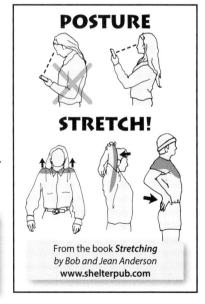

POSTURE

STRETCH!

From the book **Stretching**
by Bob and Jean Anderson
www.shelterpub.com

PHONE STRETCHES (SITTING)

APPROXIMATELY 1 MINUTE

- Do these whenever you need a break, or feel stiff.
- You needn't do all of these.
- Even one stretch can make a difference.
- Breathe.
- Stretch by the *feel*. If you do this, you'll develop body awareness: getting in touch with different parts of your body.

- Take a walk. Do something to get your blood circulating.
- After you finish the stretches, bring your phone up to eye level. Practice this often, and you'll develop a better habit.

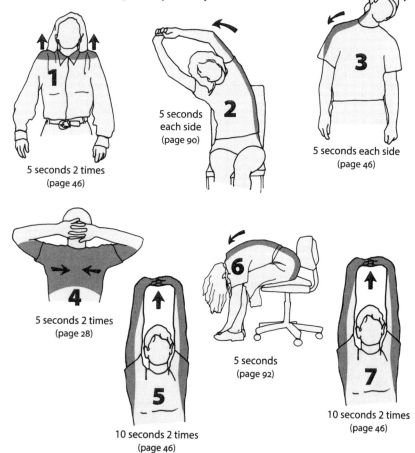

1 — 5 seconds 2 times (page 46)

2 — 5 seconds each side (page 90)

3 — 5 seconds each side (page 46)

4 — 5 seconds 2 times (page 28)

5 — 10 seconds 2 times (page 46)

6 — 5 seconds (page 92)

7 — 10 seconds 2 times (page 46)

Stretching: Pocket Book Edition © 2021 by Bob & Jean Anderson. Shelter Publications, Inc.

PHONE STRETCHES (STANDING)

APPROXIMATELY 1½ MINUTES

- Stretch until you feel a bit of tension in your muscles.
- Hold it until you relax a bit.
- Then push gently a little farther.
- Concentrate on how your muscles and tendons feel.

- The "no pain, no gain" principle does not apply to stretching.
- Breathe slowly and rhythmically.
- Practice bringing your phone up to eye level.

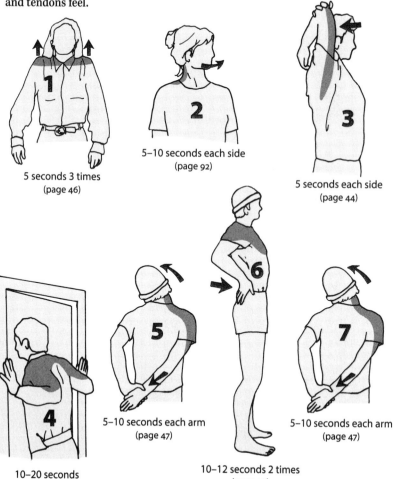

1

5 seconds 3 times
(page 46)

2

5–10 seconds each side
(page 92)

3

5 seconds each side
(page 44)

4

10–20 seconds
(page 47)

5

5–10 seconds each arm
(page 47)

6

10–12 seconds 2 times
(page 46)

7

5–10 seconds each arm
(page 47)

The Importance of Exercise

Stretching and good posture are not the only ways to counteract problems from smartphone usage, or "tech neck." Exercise increases your heart rate, sends blood to muscles, lubricates joints, and flushes out toxins that are causing pain.

Planning Plan to make exercise a part of your daily life, not just something you do at the end of the day — if you have time. Getting fit doesn't happen without planning, so you need a realistic plan for exercise to become an integral part of your life.

Make it a priority. Doing this will shape your future. Physical activity will become a priority centered around enjoyment, accomplishment, and improvement.

Be consistent. It takes longer to get into shape than it does to get out of shape. If you go a few days without exercise, don't worry; just don't go weeks or months without regular activity.

Stick with your routine. Getting fit doesn't happen by chance or without effort. It happens over time, with patience and a reasonable plan.

Learn an activity. Walking, hiking, running, cycling, swimming, weight training, etc. *Look at the list of activities on page 155.* You can google proper techniques/training for any activity you are interested in.

Take it easy. Don't overdo it when you begin. Start with a little activity, then *gradually* build it up over the year.

Rest is a very important part of getting the most out of exercise. Build rest days into your weekly plan. Rest helps prevent injuries, makes you stronger, and revitalizes the mind.

Staying hydrated improves physical and mental function, increases endurance, and helps the functioning of vital internal organs (heart, lungs, kidneys, etc.). Staying hydrated makes exercise easier and more enjoyable.

Elevate your feet every day.

Massage Get a massage as often as possible. *(See the massage body tools on pp. 228–229.)*

Staying in shape all year round will allow you to be prepared to do other activities such as vacuuming, washing the car, snow shoveling, gardening, cleaning house. Being in shape (staying strong, agile, and flexible) by regularly exercising and stretching will make it possible to do those activities more aerobically and safely.

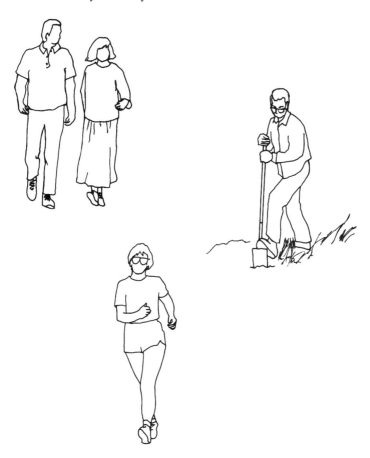

STRETCHING ROUTINES
Sports and Activities

In this section are stretching routines for sports and activities, arranged in alphabetical order.

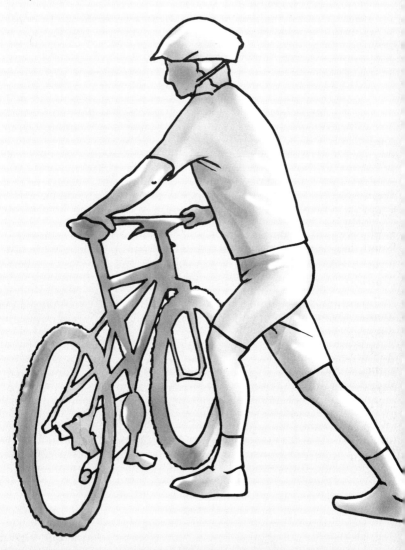

Each time you do a stretch for the first time, read the *specific* instructions for that stretch. (See the page reference under each stretch.) After you follow the instructions a few times, you'll know how to do each stretch correctly. From then on, simply look at the drawings.

Warming up: For the more vigorous sports (running, football, etc.), I recommend that you do a short warm-up before stretching (jogging for 3–5 minutes with an exaggerated arm swing, for example). See p. 14, *Warming Up and Cooling Down*.

To teachers and coaches: These routines can serve as guidelines. You can add or subtract stretches to meet specific needs and time allotments.

Note: Be sure to read *How To Stretch* on pp. 12–13 before you do these routines.

APPROXIMATELY 4 MINUTES

Do a mild warm-up of 2–3 minutes before stretching.

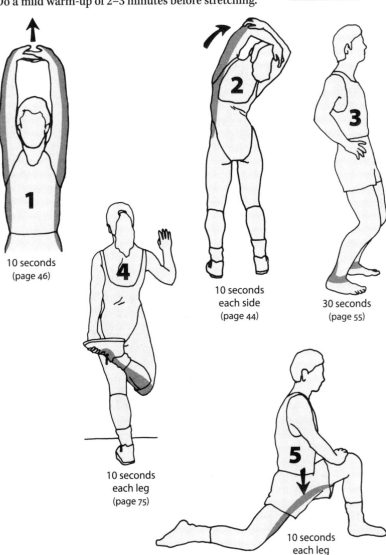

10 seconds
(page 46)

10 seconds
each side
(page 44)

30 seconds
(page 55)

10 seconds
each leg
(page 75)

10 seconds
each leg
(page 53)

Stretching: Pocket Book Edition © 2021 by Bob and Jean Anderson. Shelter Publications, Inc.

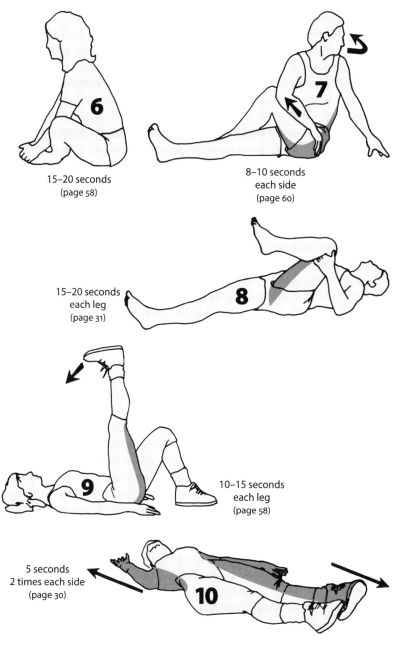

15–20 seconds
(page 58)

8–10 seconds
each side
(page 60)

15–20 seconds
each leg
(page 31)

10–15 seconds
each leg
(page 58)

5 seconds
2 times each side
(page 30)

Stretching: Pocket Book Edition © 2021 by Bob and Jean Anderson. Shelter Publications, Inc.

APPROXIMATELY 4 MINUTES

Warm up with 2–3 minutes of walking before stretching.

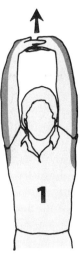

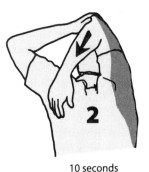

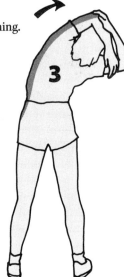

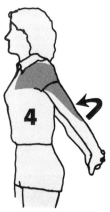

1

10–15 seconds
(page 46)

2

10 seconds
each arm
(page 44)

3

8–10 seconds
each side
(page 44)

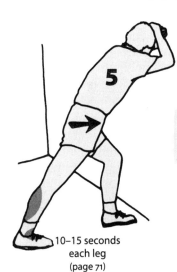

4

10–15 seconds
2 times
(page 47)

5

10–15 seconds
each leg
(page 71)

Mini-routine:
3, 4, 6, 7, 9
Approx. 2 min.

Stretching: Pocket Book Edition © 2021 by Bob and Jean Anderson. Shelter Publications, Inc.

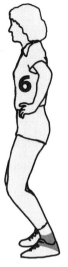

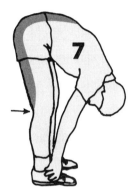

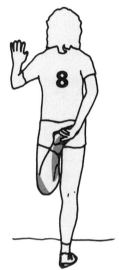

6

15–30 seconds
(page 55)

7

15–20 seconds
(page 54)

8

10–15 seconds
each leg
(page 75)

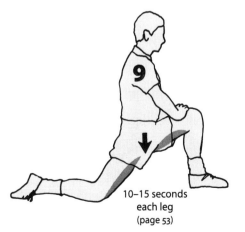

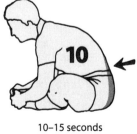

9

10–15 seconds
each leg
(page 53)

10

10–15 seconds
(page 58)

APPROXIMATELY 5 MINUTES

Jog around the baseball field once before stretching.

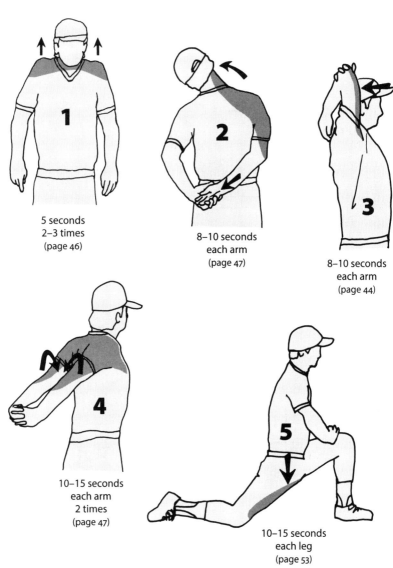

1

5 seconds
2–3 times
(page 46)

2

8–10 seconds
each arm
(page 47)

3

8–10 seconds
each arm
(page 44)

4

10–15 seconds
each arm
2 times
(page 47)

5

10–15 seconds
each leg
(page 53)

    Stretching: Pocket Book Edition © 2021 by Bob and Jean Anderson. Shelter Publications, Inc.

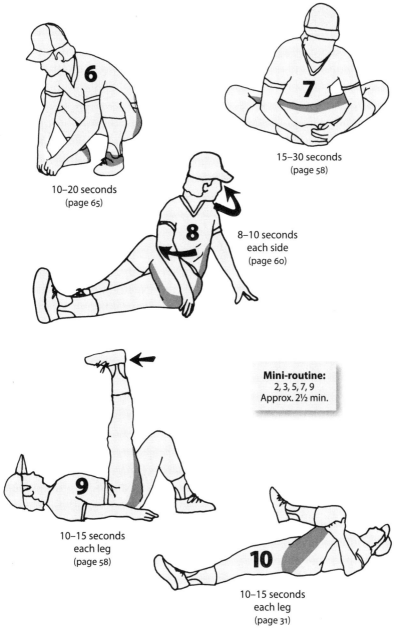

6

10–20 seconds
(page 65)

7

15–30 seconds
(page 58)

8

8–10 seconds
each side
(page 60)

9

10–15 seconds
each leg
(page 58)

Mini-routine:
2, 3, 5, 7, 9
Approx. 2½ min.

10

10–15 seconds
each leg
(page 31)

APPROXIMATELY 4 MINUTES

Warm up by jogging for 3–5 minutes before stretching.

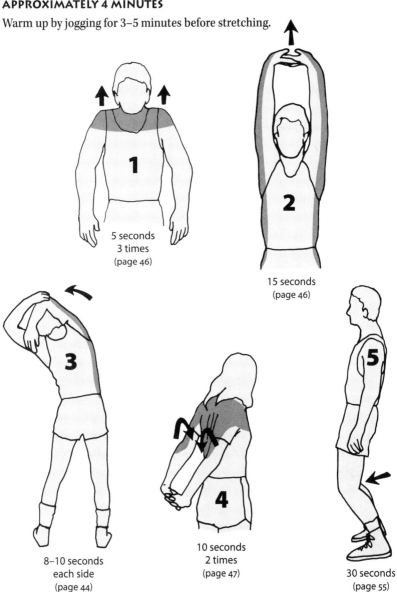

1
5 seconds
3 times
(page 46)

2
15 seconds
(page 46)

3
8–10 seconds
each side
(page 44)

4
10 seconds
2 times
(page 47)

5
30 seconds
(page 55)

Stretching: Pocket Book Edition © 2021 by Bob and Jean Anderson. Shelter Publications, Inc.

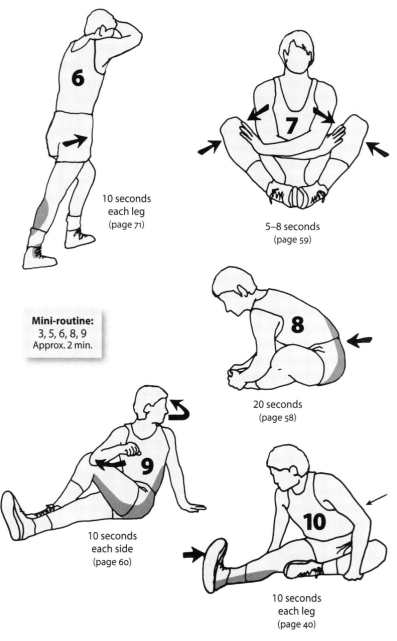

6

10 seconds
each leg
(page 71)

7

5–8 seconds
(page 59)

Mini-routine:
3, 5, 6, 8, 9
Approx. 2 min.

8

20 seconds
(page 58)

9

10 seconds
each side
(page 60)

10

10 seconds
each leg
(page 40)

APPROXIMATELY 3 MINUTES

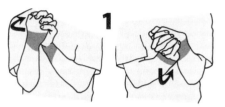

Rotate 10 times
each direction
(page 88)

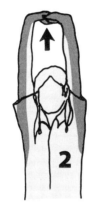

15 seconds
(page 46)

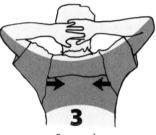

5 seconds
2 times
(page 91)

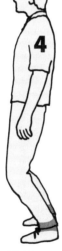

15–20 seconds
(page 55)

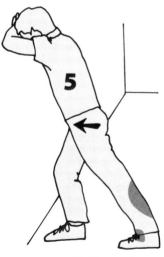

10–15 seconds
each leg
(page 71)

Stretching: Pocket Book Edition © 2021 by Bob and Jean Anderson. Shelter Publications, Inc.

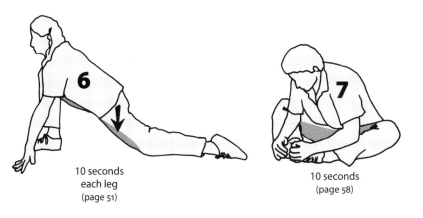

6

10 seconds
each leg
(page 51)

7

10 seconds
(page 58)

Mini-routine:
2, 6, 7, 9, 10
Approx. 1½ min.

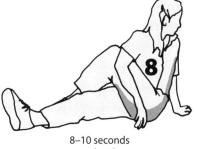

8

8–10 seconds
each side
(page 60)

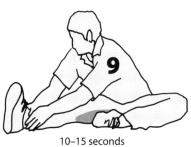

9

10–15 seconds
each leg
(page 39)

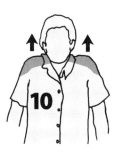

10

5 seconds
3 times
(page 46)

APPROXIMATELY 5 MINUTES

Walk for several minutes before stretching.

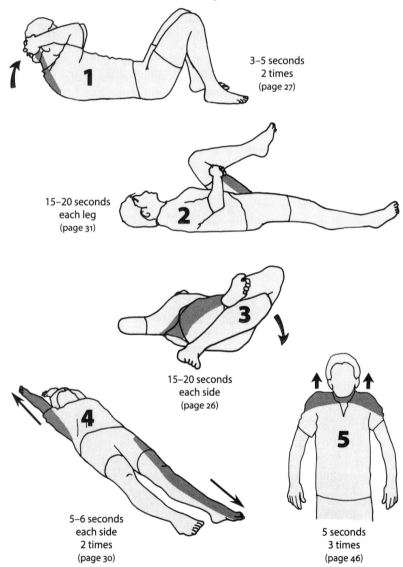

3–5 seconds
2 times
(page 27)

15–20 seconds
each leg
(page 31)

15–20 seconds
each side
(page 26)

5–6 seconds
each side
2 times
(page 30)

5 seconds
3 times
(page 46)

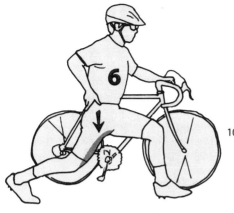

6

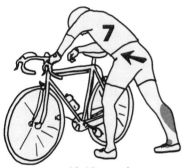

7

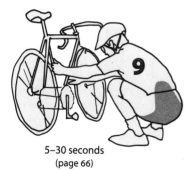

9

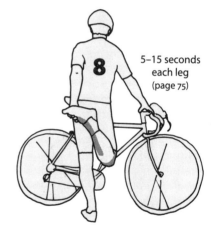

8

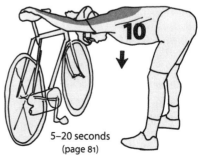

10

Mini-routine:
2, 7, 8, 9, 10
Approx. 2½ min.

10–20 seconds
each leg
(page 53)

10–15 seconds
each leg
(page 71)

5–15 seconds
each leg
(page 75)

5–30 seconds
(page 66)

5–20 seconds
(page 81)

APPROXIMATELY 4 MINUTES

Walk for 2–3 minutes before stretching.

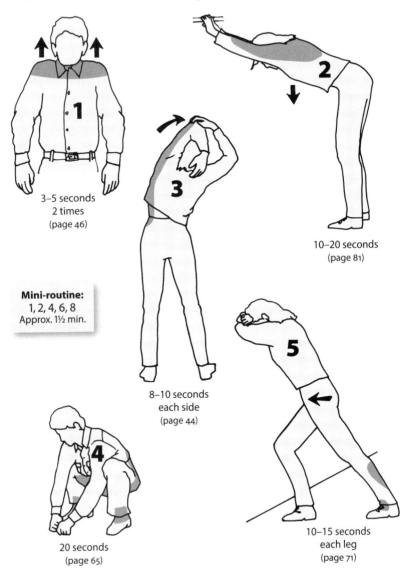

3–5 seconds
2 times
(page 46)

10–20 seconds
(page 81)

Mini-routine:
1, 2, 4, 6, 8
Approx. 1½ min.

8–10 seconds
each side
(page 44)

20 seconds
(page 65)

10–15 seconds
each leg
(page 71)

Stretching: Pocket Book Edition © 2021 by Bob and Jean Anderson. Shelter Publications, Inc.

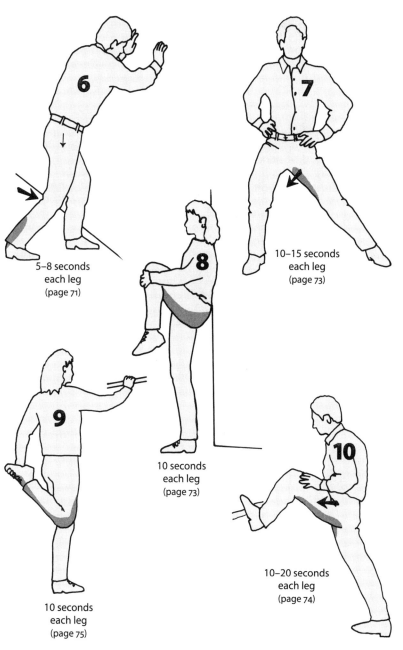

6

5–8 seconds
each leg
(page 71)

7

10–15 seconds
each leg
(page 73)

8

10 seconds
each leg
(page 73)

9

10 seconds
each leg
(page 75)

10

10–20 seconds
each leg
(page 74)

APPROXIMATELY 5 MINUTES

Warm up for 4–5 minutes before stretching.

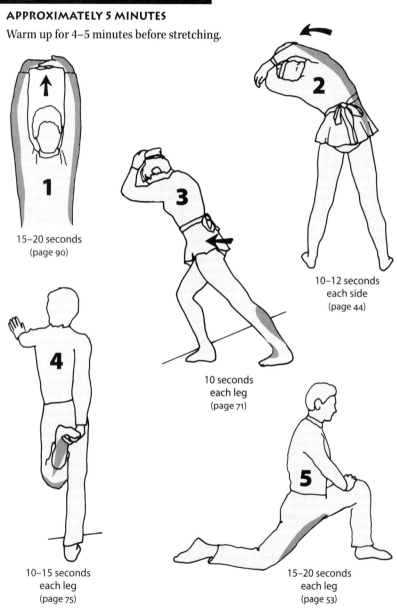

1

15–20 seconds
(page 90)

2

10–12 seconds
each side
(page 44)

3

10 seconds
each leg
(page 71)

4

10–15 seconds
each leg
(page 75)

5

15–20 seconds
each leg
(page 53)

Stretching: Pocket Book Edition © 2021 by Bob and Jean Anderson. Shelter Publications, Inc.

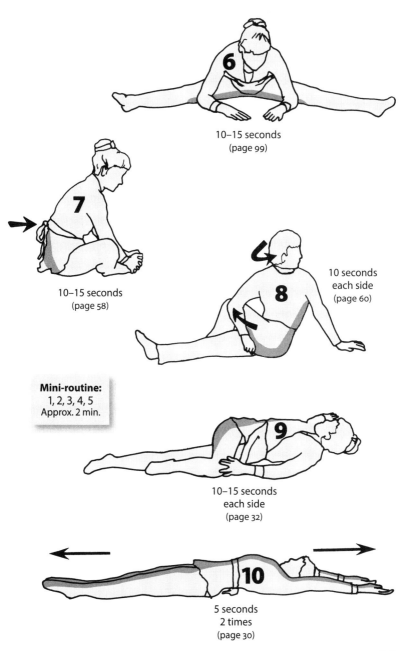

6

10–15 seconds
(page 99)

7

10–15 seconds
(page 58)

8

10 seconds
each side
(page 60)

Mini-routine:
1, 2, 3, 4, 5
Approx. 2 min.

9

10–15 seconds
each side
(page 32)

10

5 seconds
2 times
(page 30)

Stretching: Pocket Book Edition © 2021 by Bob and Jean Anderson. Shelter Publications, Inc.

APPROXIMATELY 4 MINUTES

Jog around the football field before stretching.

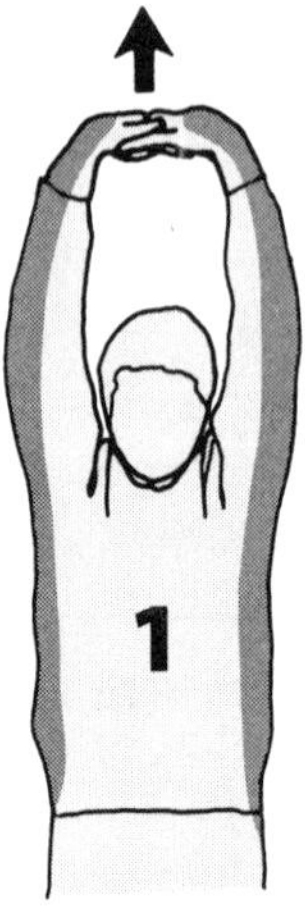

1

10 seconds
2 times
(page 46)

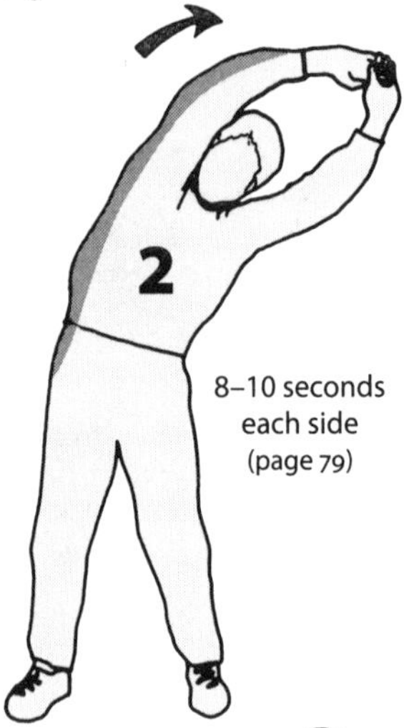

2

8–10 seconds
each side
(page 79)

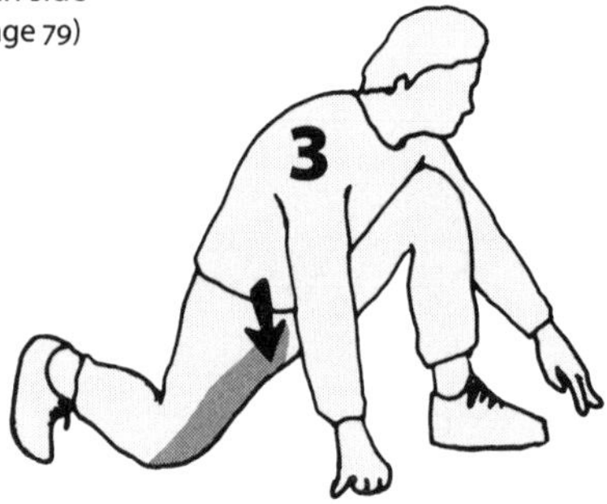

3

10–15 seconds
each leg
(page 51)

Mini-routine:
1, 2, 3, 8, 10
Approx. 2 min.

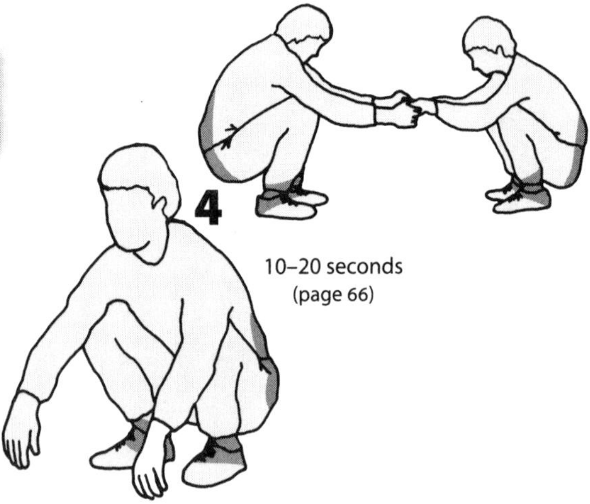

4

10–20 seconds
(page 66)

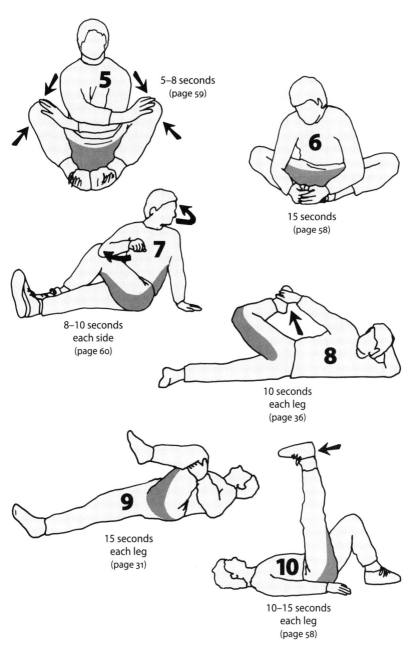

5 5–8 seconds
(page 59)

6 15 seconds
(page 58)

7 8–10 seconds
each side
(page 60)

8 10 seconds
each leg
(page 36)

9 15 seconds
each leg
(page 31)

10 10–15 seconds
each leg
(page 58)

APPROXIMATELY 4 MINUTES

Walk for several minutes before stretching.

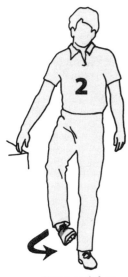

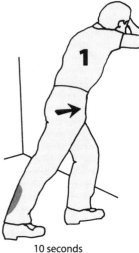

10 seconds
each leg
(page 71)

Rotate each foot
10–15 times
(page 71)

Mini-routine:
1, 3, 8, 9, 10
Approx. 2 min.

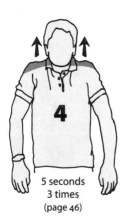

15–20 seconds
(page 55)

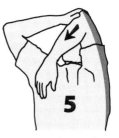

5 seconds
3 times
(page 46)

10 seconds
each arm
2 times
(page 44)

Stretching: Pocket Book Edition © 2021 by Bob and Jean Anderson. Shelter Publications, Inc.

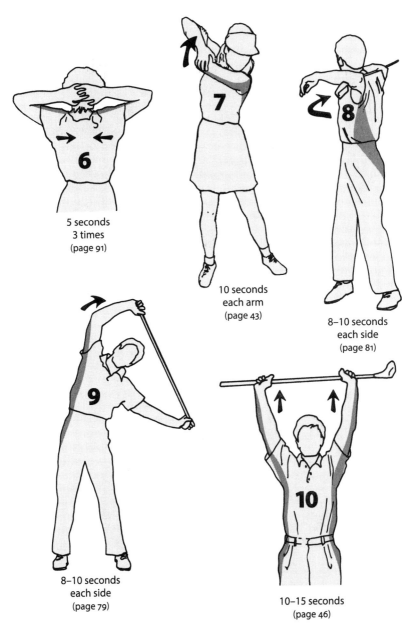

5 seconds
3 times
(page 91)

10 seconds
each arm
(page 43)

8–10 seconds
each side
(page 81)

8–10 seconds
each side
(page 79)

10–15 seconds
(page 46)

APPROXIMATELY 6 MINUTES

Warm up for 4–5 minutes by walking or jogging before stretching.

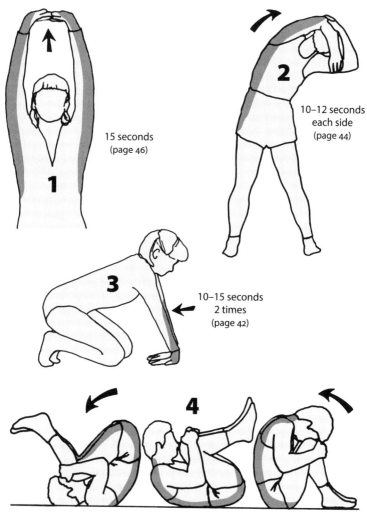

15 seconds
(page 46)

10–12 seconds
each side
(page 44)

10–15 seconds
2 times
(page 42)

Gently roll
6–12 times
(page 63)

Stretching: Pocket Book Edition © 2021 by Bob and Jean Anderson. Shelter Publications, Inc.

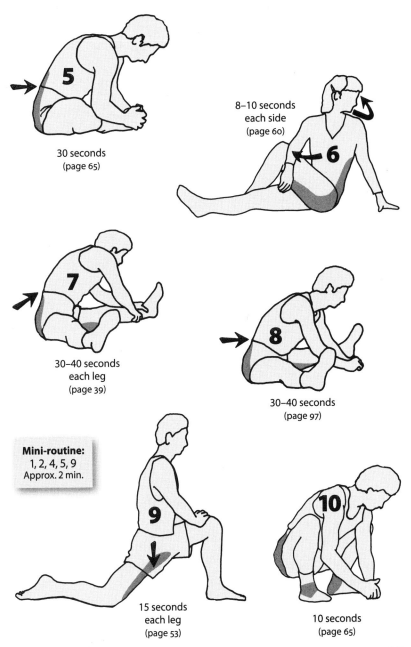

5
30 seconds
(page 65)

8–10 seconds
each side
(page 60)

6

7
30–40 seconds
each leg
(page 39)

8
30–40 seconds
(page 97)

Mini-routine:
1, 2, 4, 5, 9
Approx. 2 min.

9
15 seconds
each leg
(page 53)

10
10 seconds
(page 65)

APPROXIMATELY 4 MINUTES

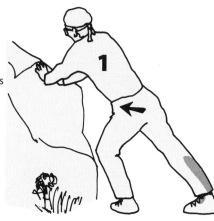

10–15 seconds
each leg
(page 71)

1

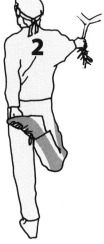

2

10–15 seconds
each leg
(page 75)

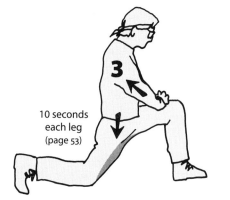

3

10 seconds
each leg
(page 53)

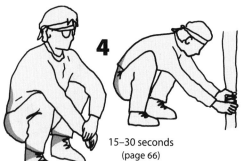

4

15–30 seconds
(page 66)

> **Mini-routine:**
> 1, 2, 3, 4, 5
> Approx. 2½ min.

Stretching: Pocket Book Edition © 2021 by Bob and Jean Anderson. Shelter Publications, Inc.

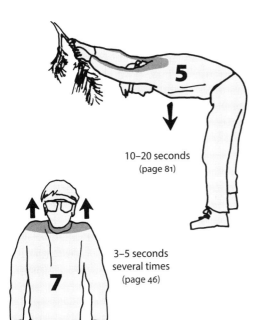

10–20 seconds
(page 81)

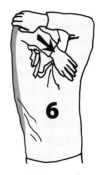

8–10 seconds
each arm
(page 44)

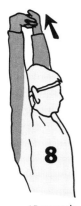

3–5 seconds
several times
(page 46)

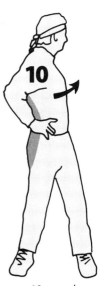

15 seconds
(page 46)

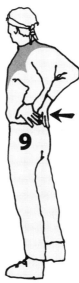

10 seconds
2 times
(page 46)

10 seconds
each side
(page 81)

APPROXIMATELY 4 MINUTES

Warm up by walking or riding a stationary bike for 2–4 minutes before stretching.

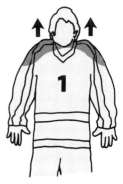

1

5 seconds
3 times
(page 46)

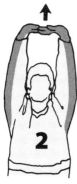

2

5–10 seconds
(page 46)

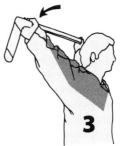

3

10–15 seconds
(page 87)

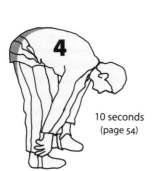

4

10 seconds
(page 54)

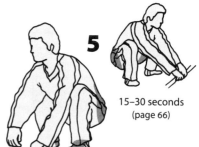

5

15–30 seconds
(page 66)

Stretching: Pocket Book Edition © 2021 by Bob and Jean Anderson. Shelter Publications, Inc.

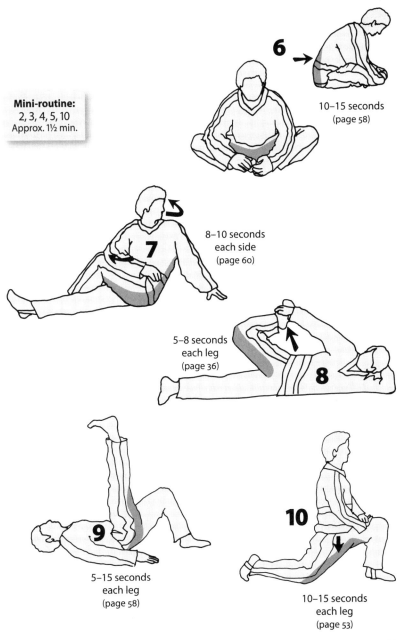

Mini-routine:
2, 3, 4, 5, 10
Approx. 1½ min.

6

10–15 seconds
(page 58)

7

8–10 seconds
each side
(page 60)

8

5–8 seconds
each leg
(page 36)

9

5–15 seconds
each leg
(page 58)

10

10–15 seconds
each leg
(page 53)

APPROXIMATELY 4 MINUTES

Walk for several minutes before stretching.

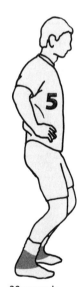

10 seconds
(page 46)

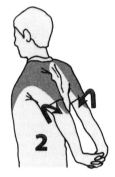

15 seconds
(page 47)

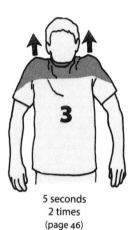

5 seconds
2 times
(page 46)

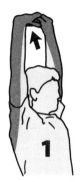

10 seconds
each side
(page 44)

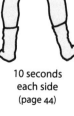

30 seconds
(page 55)

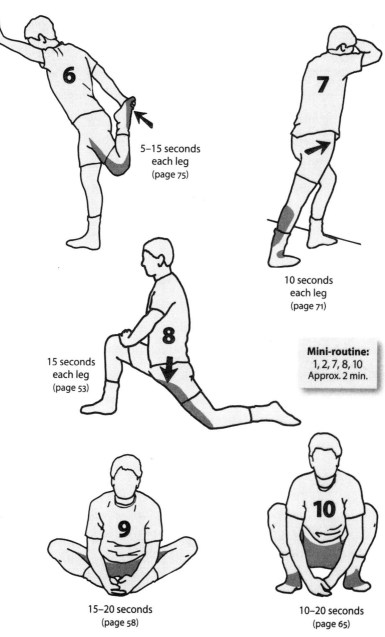

6 5–15 seconds
each leg
(page 75)

7 10 seconds
each leg
(page 71)

8 15 seconds
each leg
(page 53)

Mini-routine:
1, 2, 7, 8, 10
Approx. 2 min.

9 15–20 seconds
(page 58)

10 10–20 seconds
(page 65)

APPROXIMATELY 3 MINUTES

Walk for several minutes before stretching.

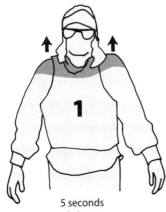

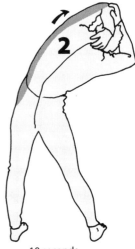

5 seconds
3 times
(page 46)

10 seconds
each side
(page 44)

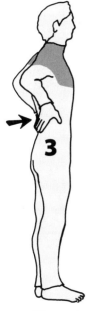

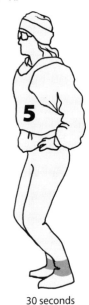

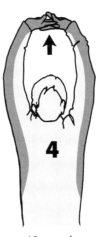

10 seconds
(page 46)

15 seconds
(page 46)

30 seconds
(page 55)

Stretching: Pocket Book Edition © 2021 by Bob and Jean Anderson. Shelter Publications, Inc.

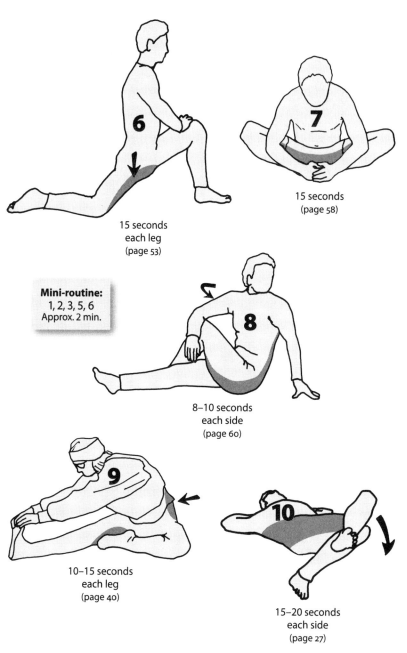

6

15 seconds
each leg
(page 53)

7

15 seconds
(page 58)

Mini-routine:
1, 2, 3, 5, 6
Approx. 2 min.

8

8–10 seconds
each side
(page 60)

9

10–15 seconds
each leg
(page 40)

10

15–20 seconds
each side
(page 27)

APPROXIMATELY 4 MINUTES

Note: These stretches are not intended to replace your traditional routine, but can be used for improvement of overall flexibility. They should be preceded by a good warm-up.

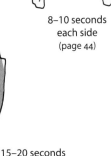

8–10 seconds
each side
(page 44)

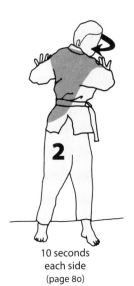

10 seconds
each side
(page 80)

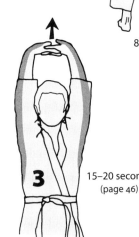

15–20 seconds
(page 46)

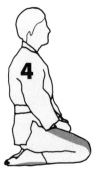

20–30 seconds
(page 49)

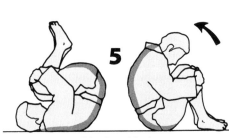

Roll back and forth
10–12 times
(page 63)

Stretching: Pocket Book Edition © 2021 by Bob and Jean Anderson. Shelter Publications, Inc.

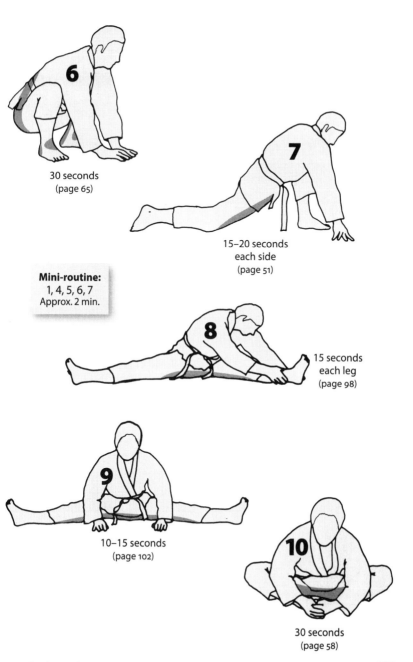

6

30 seconds
(page 65)

7

15–20 seconds
each side
(page 51)

Mini-routine:
1, 4, 5, 6, 7
Approx. 2 min.

8

15 seconds
each leg
(page 98)

9

10–15 seconds
(page 102)

10

30 seconds
(page 58)

APPROXIMATELY 4 MINUTES

Walk around for several minutes before stretching.

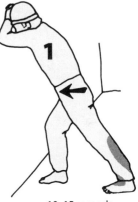

10–15 seconds
each leg
(page 71)

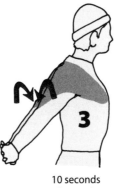

15 seconds
(page 46)

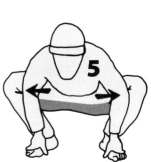

10 seconds
(page 47)

Mini-routine:
1, 3, 4, 5, 6
Approx. 2 min.

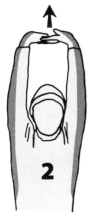

8–10 seconds
each side
(page 44)

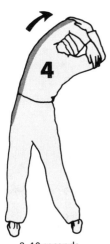

10 seconds
(page 66)

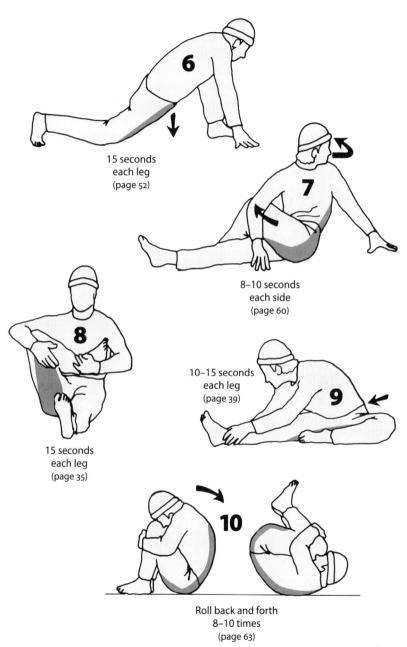

6

15 seconds
each leg
(page 52)

7

8–10 seconds
each side
(page 60)

8

15 seconds
each leg
(page 35)

9

10–15 seconds
each leg
(page 39)

10

Roll back and forth
8–10 times
(page 63)

APPROXIMATELY 4 MINUTES

Warm up by riding or walking for 3–5 minutes before stretching.

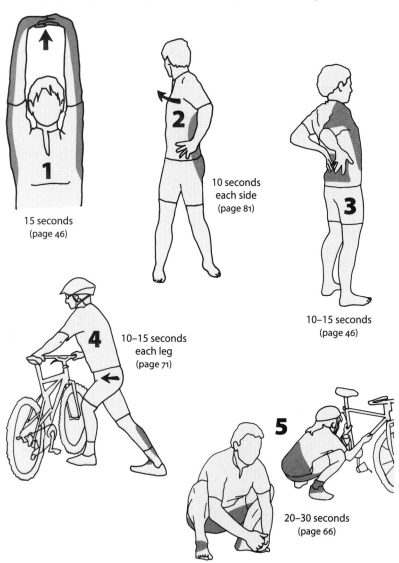

1 15 seconds (page 46)

2 10 seconds each side (page 81)

3 10–15 seconds (page 46)

4 10–15 seconds each leg (page 71)

5 20–30 seconds (page 66)

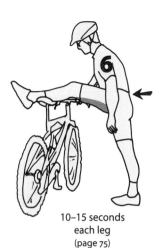

10–15 seconds
each leg
(page 75)

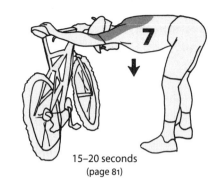

15–20 seconds
(page 81)

Mini-routine:
4, 5, 6, 7, 10
Approx. 2 min.

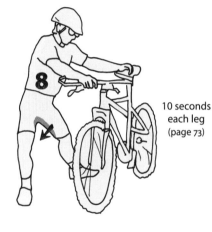

10 seconds
each leg
(page 73)

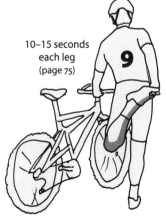

10–15 seconds
each leg
(page 75)

10–15 seconds
each leg
(page 53)

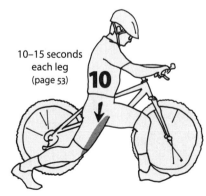

APPROXIMATELY 5 MINUTES

Warm up for 2–4 minutes before stretching.

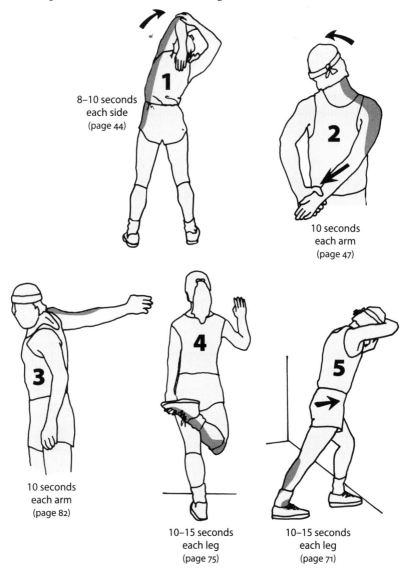

8–10 seconds
each side
(page 44)

10 seconds
each arm
(page 47)

10 seconds
each arm
(page 82)

10–15 seconds
each leg
(page 75)

10–15 seconds
each leg
(page 71)

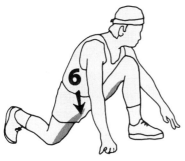

10–20 seconds
each leg
(page 51)

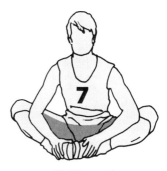

15–20 seconds
(page 58)

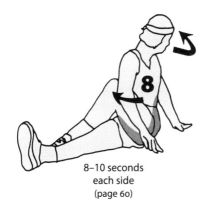

8–10 seconds
each side
(page 60)

Mini-routine:
2, 3, 5, 6, 10
Approx. 2½ min.

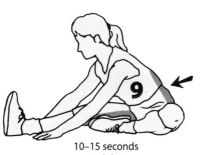

10–15 seconds
each leg
(page 39)

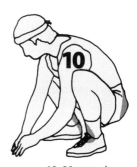

10–20 seconds
(page 65)

APPROXIMATELY 4 MINUTES

Walk for several minutes before stretching.

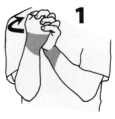

Rotate wrists
10 times clockwise
and counterclockwise
(page 88)

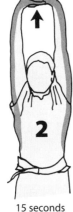

15 seconds
(page 46)

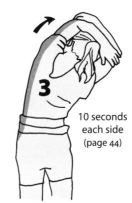

10 seconds
each side
(page 44)

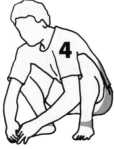

15–30 seconds
(page 65)

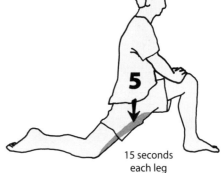

15 seconds
each leg
(page 53)

Stretching: Pocket Book Edition © 2021 by Bob and Jean Anderson. Shelter Publications, Inc.

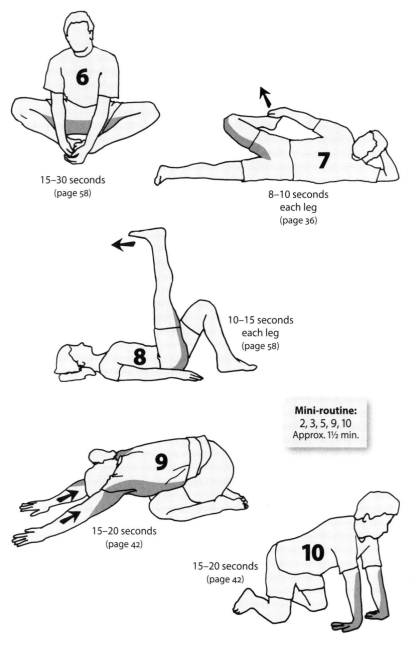

6

15–30 seconds
(page 58)

7

8–10 seconds
each leg
(page 36)

8

10–15 seconds
each leg
(page 58)

Mini-routine:
2, 3, 5, 9, 10
Approx. 1½ min.

9

15–20 seconds
(page 42)

15–20 seconds
(page 42)

10

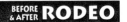
APPROXIMATELY 2 MINUTES

Walk for several minutes before stretching.

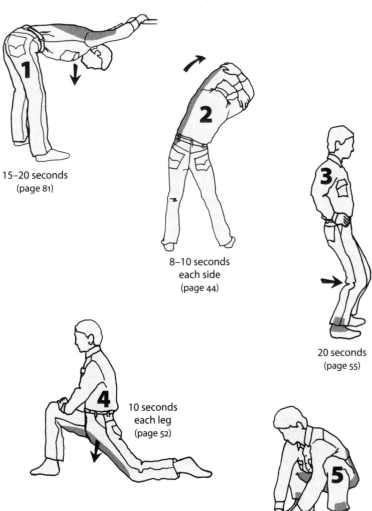

15–20 seconds
(page 81)

8–10 seconds
each side
(page 44)

20 seconds
(page 55)

10 seconds
each leg
(page 52)

20 seconds
(page 65)

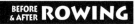
APPROXIMATELY 2 MINUTES

Warm up by moving for 3–5 minutes before stretching.

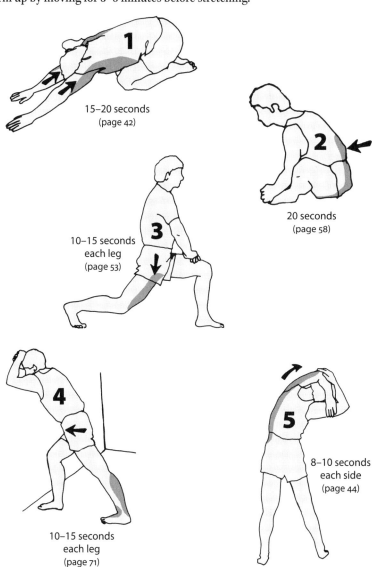

1 15–20 seconds
(page 42)

2 20 seconds
(page 58)

3 10–15 seconds
each leg
(page 53)

4 10–15 seconds
each leg
(page 71)

5 8–10 seconds
each side
(page 44)

APPROXIMATELY 3 MINUTES

Warm up by jogging for 3–5 minutes before stretching.

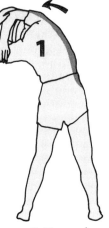

8–10 seconds
each side
(page 44)

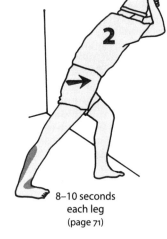

8–10 seconds
each leg
(page 71)

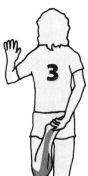

10–15 seconds
each leg
(page 75)

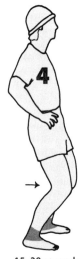

15–30 seconds
(page 55)

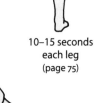

15 seconds
each leg
(page 51)

Stretching: Pocket Book Edition © 2021 by Bob and Jean Anderson. Shelter Publications, Inc.

APPROXIMATELY 2 MINUTES

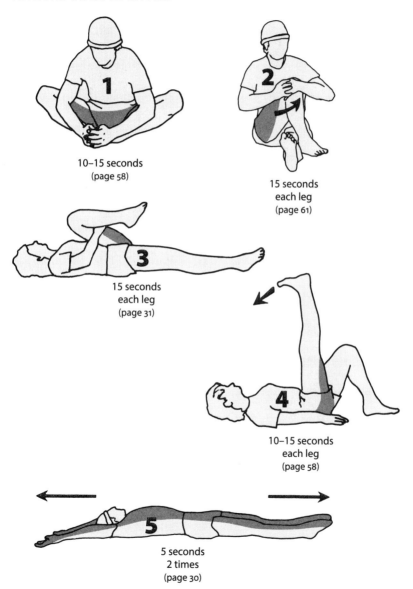

1

10–15 seconds
(page 58)

2

15 seconds
each leg
(page 61)

3

15 seconds
each leg
(page 31)

4

10–15 seconds
each leg
(page 58)

5

5 seconds
2 times
(page 30)

APPROXIMATELY 2 MINUTES

Warm up by walking for several minutes with a big arm swing before stretching.

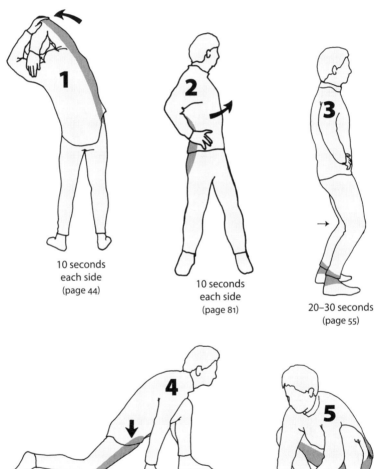

1

10 seconds
each side
(page 44)

2

10 seconds
each side
(page 81)

3

20–30 seconds
(page 55)

4

10–15 seconds
each leg
(page 51)

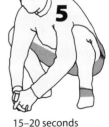

5

15–20 seconds
(page 65)

Stretching: Pocket Book Edition © 2021 by Bob and Jean Anderson. Shelter Publications, Inc.

APPROXIMATELY 2 MINUTES

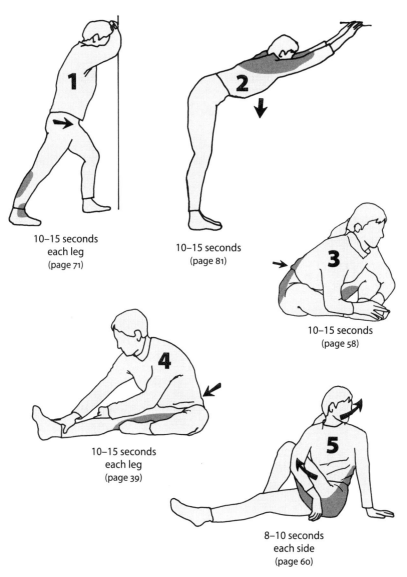

10–15 seconds
each leg
(page 71)

10–15 seconds
(page 81)

10–15 seconds
(page 58)

10–15 seconds
each leg
(page 39)

8–10 seconds
each side
(page 60)

APPROXIMATELY 2 MINUTES

Walk for 2–3 minutes.

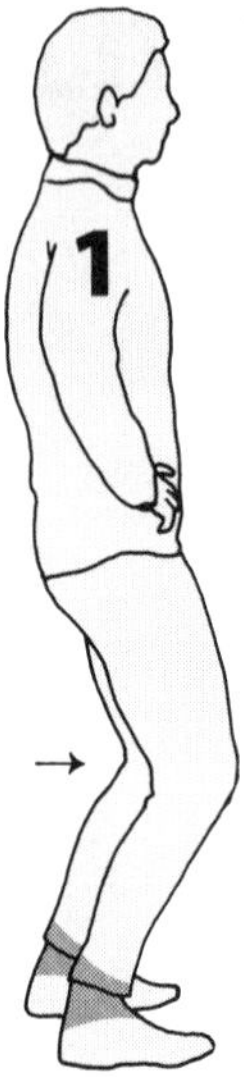

1

30 seconds
(page 55)

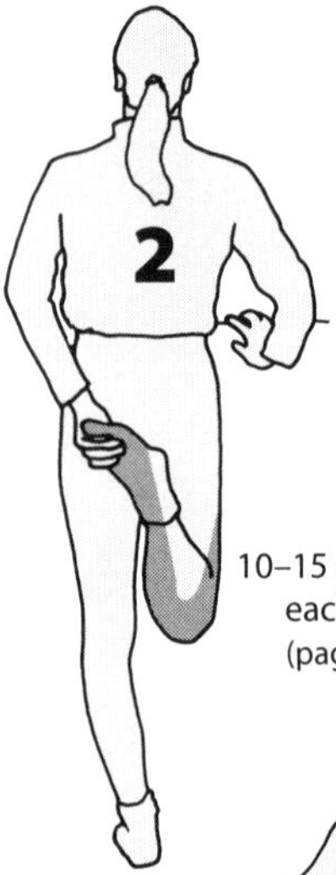

2

10–15 seconds
each leg
(page 75)

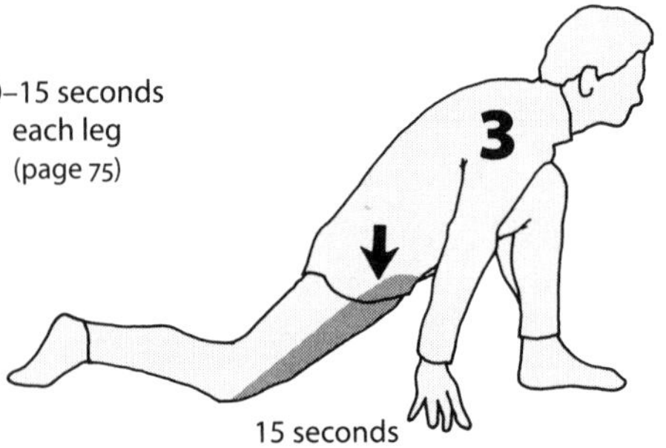

3

15 seconds
each leg
(page 51)

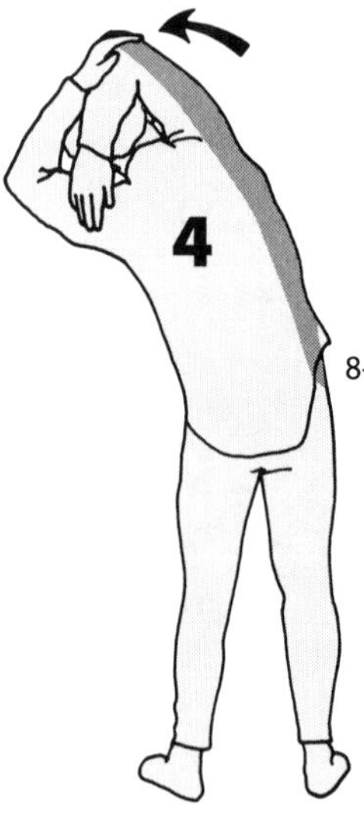

4

8–10 seconds
each side
(page 44)

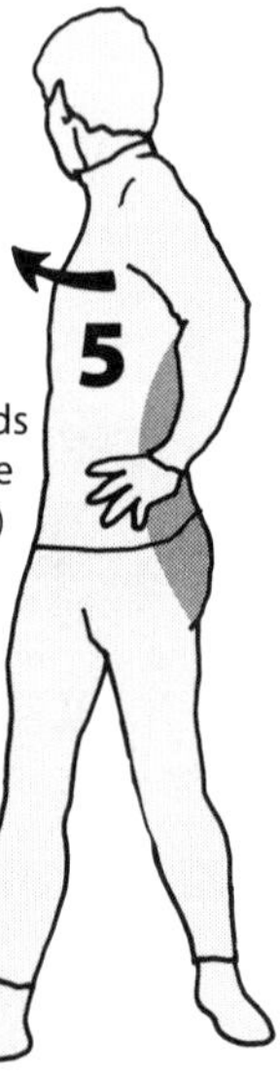

5

10 seconds
each side
(page 81)

Stretching: Pocket Book Edition © 2021 by Bob and Jean Anderson. Shelter Publications, Inc.

APPROXIMATELY 2 MINUTES

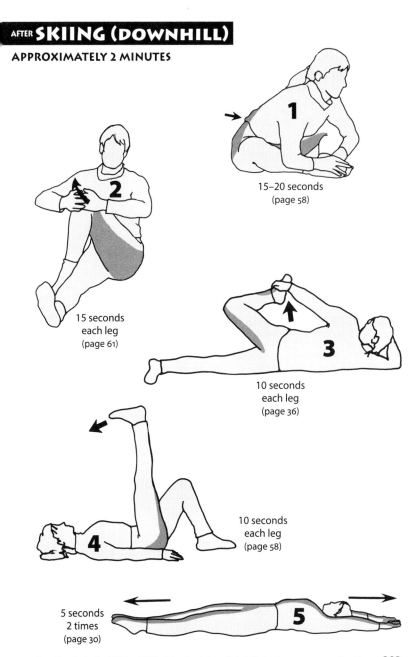

15–20 seconds
(page 58)

15 seconds
each leg
(page 61)

10 seconds
each leg
(page 36)

10 seconds
each leg
(page 58)

5 seconds
2 times
(page 30)

APPROXIMATELY 3 MINUTES

Walk for several minutes before stretching.

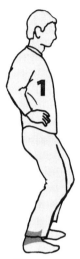

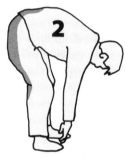

10–15 seconds
(page 54)

30 seconds
(page 55)

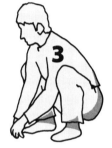

10–15 seconds
(page 65)

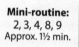

Mini-routine:
2, 3, 4, 8, 9
Approx. 1½ min.

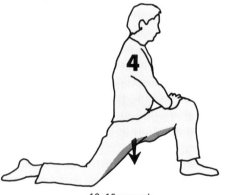

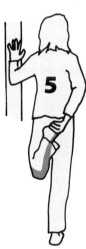

10–15 seconds
each leg
(page 53)

10 seconds
each leg
(page 75)

Stretching: Pocket Book Edition © 2021 by Bob and Jean Anderson. Shelter Publications, Inc.

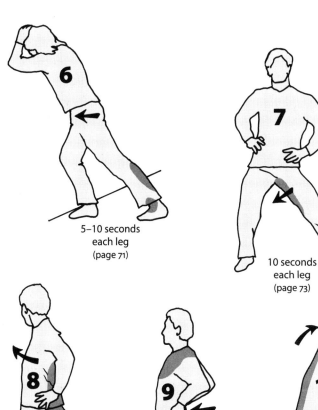

5–10 seconds
each leg
(page 71)

10 seconds
each leg
(page 73)

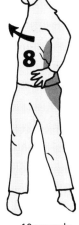

10 seconds
each side
(page 81)

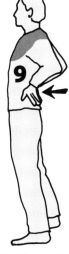

10–15 seconds
(page 46)

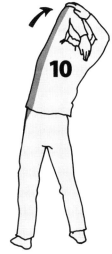

8–10 seconds
each side
(page 44)

APPROXIMATELY 2 MINUTES

Jog around the soccer field before stretching.

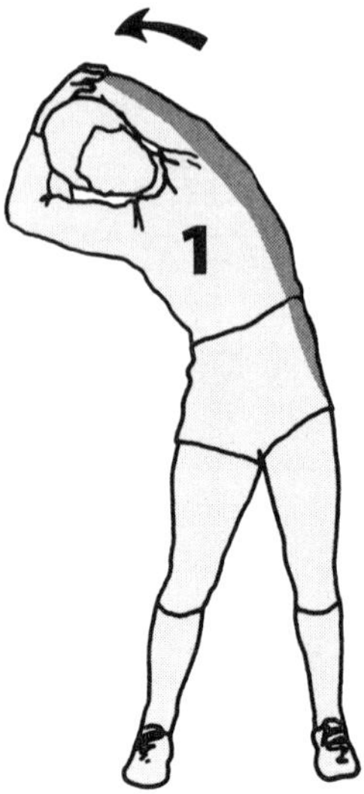

1

8–10 seconds
each side
(page 44)

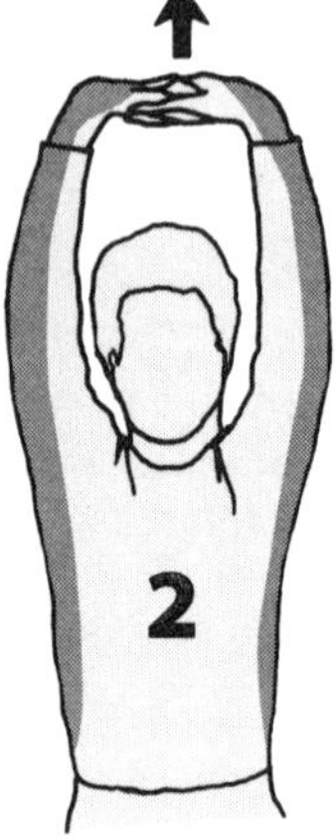

2

10–15 seconds
(page 46)

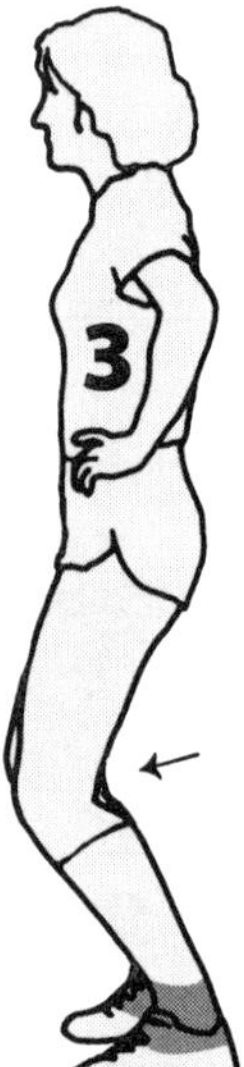

3

20–30 seconds
(page 55)

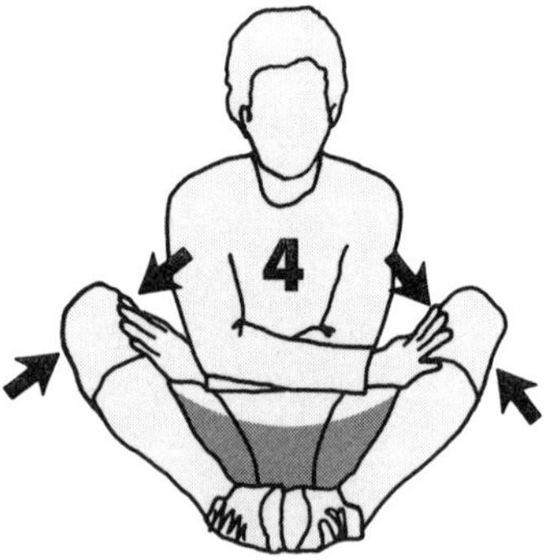

4

5–8 seconds
(page 59)

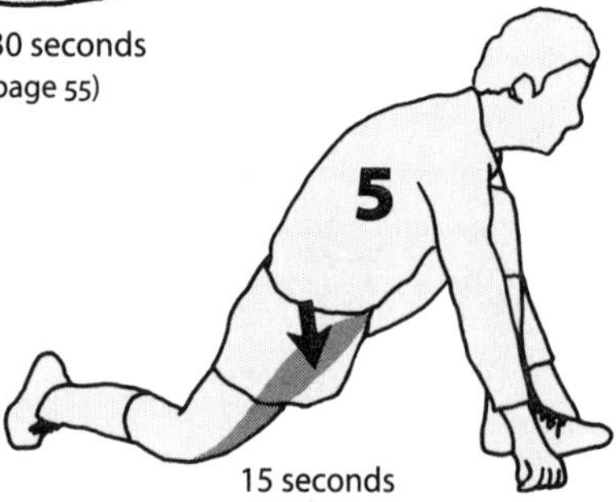

5

15 seconds
each leg
(page 52)

APPROXIMATELY 2 MINUTES

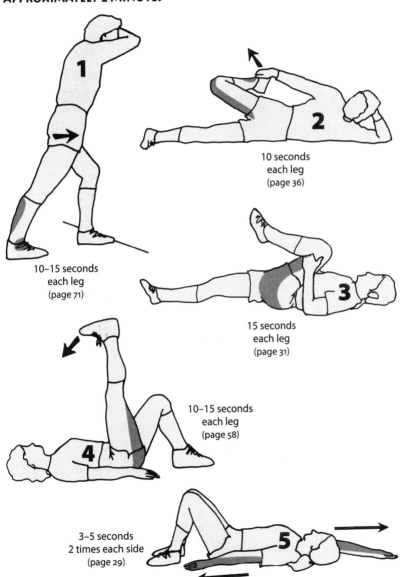

1 10–15 seconds
each leg
(page 71)

2 10 seconds
each leg
(page 36)

3 15 seconds
each leg
(page 31)

4 10–15 seconds
each leg
(page 58)

5 3–5 seconds
2 times each side
(page 29)

APPROXIMATELY 3 MINUTES

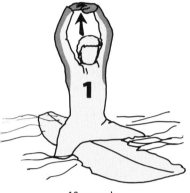

10 seconds
(page 90)

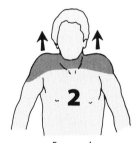

5 seconds
3 times
(page 46)

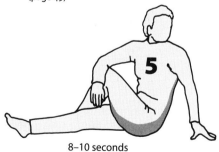

10–15 seconds
(page 49)

You can do these stretches in the water while waiting for a set: 1, 3, 4, 6, 9
Approx. 1½ min.

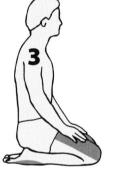

15 seconds
(page 58)

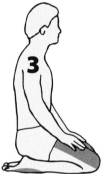

8–10 seconds
each side
(page 60)

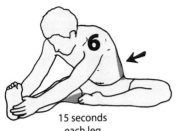

6

15 seconds
each leg
(page 39)

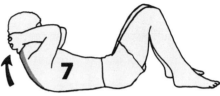

7

3–5 seconds
2 times
(page 27)

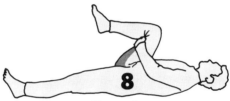

8

10 seconds
each leg
(page 31)

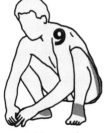

9

20–30 seconds
(page 65)

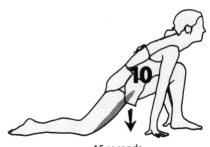

10

15 seconds
each leg
(page 51)

APPROXIMATELY 3 MINUTES

Walk with a big arm swing for 2–3 minutes before stretching.

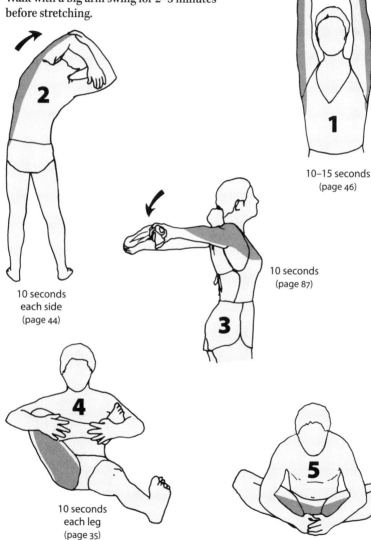

10–15 seconds
(page 46)

10 seconds
each side
(page 44)

10 seconds
(page 87)

10 seconds
each leg
(page 35)

15 seconds
(page 58)

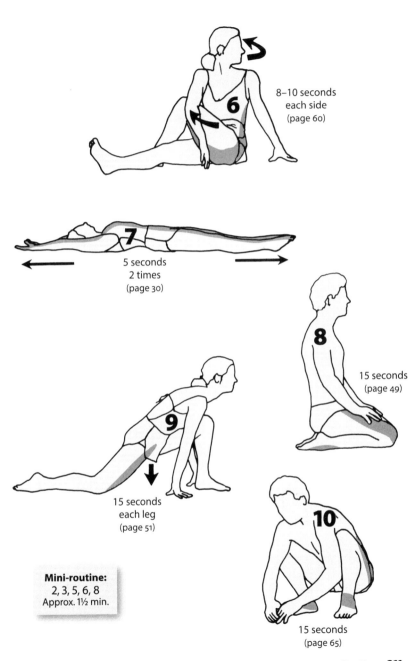

6
8–10 seconds
each side
(page 60)

7
5 seconds
2 times
(page 30)

8
15 seconds
(page 49)

9
15 seconds
each leg
(page 51)

10
15 seconds
(page 65)

Mini-routine:
2, 3, 5, 6, 8
Approx. 1½ min.

APPROXIMATELY 3 MINUTES

Walk for several minutes before stretching.

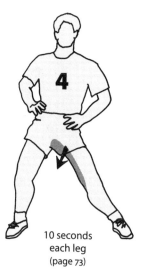

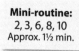

Rotate each foot
10 times
each direction
(page 71)

15 seconds
each leg
(page 71)

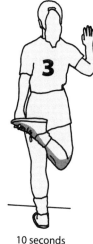

Mini-routine:
2, 3, 6, 8, 10
Approx. 1½ min.

10 seconds
each leg
(page 75)

10 seconds
each leg
(page 73)

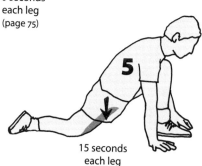

15 seconds
each leg
(page 51)

Stretching: Pocket Book Edition © 2021 by Bob and Jean Anderson. Shelter Publications, Inc.

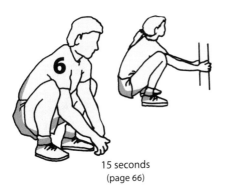

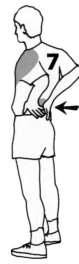

15 seconds
(page 66)

10 seconds
(page 46)

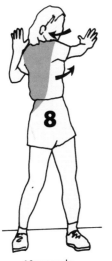

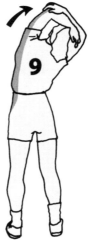

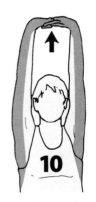

10 seconds
each side
(page 80)

8–10 seconds
each side
(page 44)

5–10 seconds
(page 46)

APPROXIMATELY 3 MINUTES

Walk or jog for several minutes before stretching.

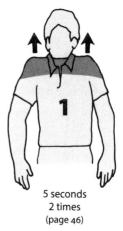

1

5 seconds
2 times
(page 46)

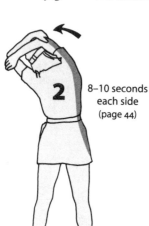

2

8–10 seconds
each side
(page 44)

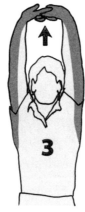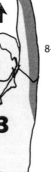

3

8–10 seconds
(page 46)

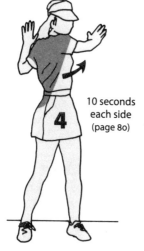

4

10 seconds
each side
(page 80)

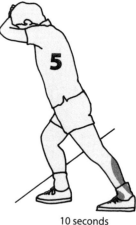

5

10 seconds
each leg
(page 71)

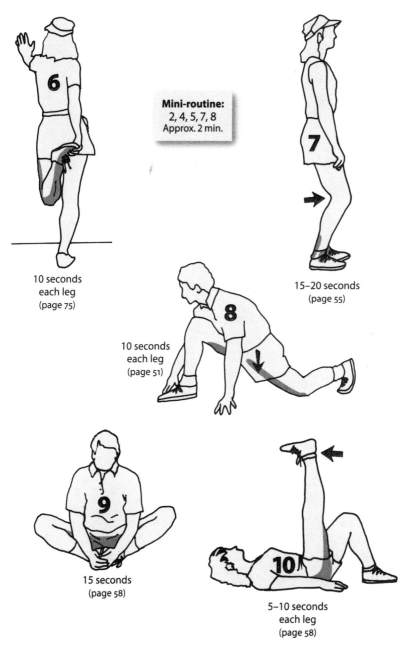

Mini-routine:
2, 4, 5, 7, 8
Approx. 2 min.

10 seconds
each leg
(page 75)

15–20 seconds
(page 55)

10 seconds
each leg
(page 51)

15 seconds
(page 58)

5–10 seconds
each leg
(page 58)

Stretching: Pocket Book Edition © 2021 by Bob and Jean Anderson. Shelter Publications, Inc.

APPROXIMATELY 4 MINUTES

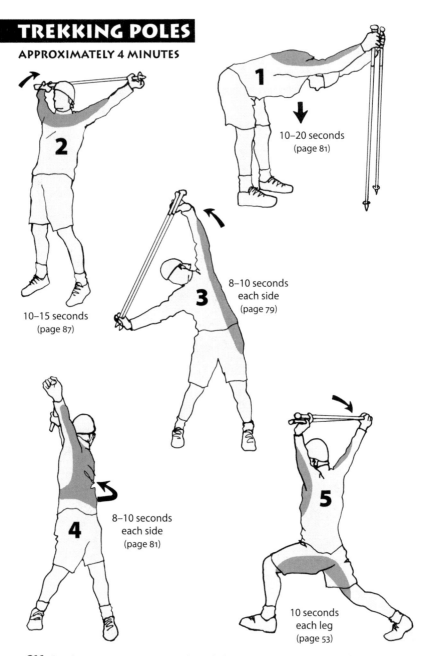

1

10–20 seconds
(page 81)

2

10–15 seconds
(page 87)

3

8–10 seconds
each side
(page 79)

4

8–10 seconds
each side
(page 81)

5

10 seconds
each leg
(page 53)

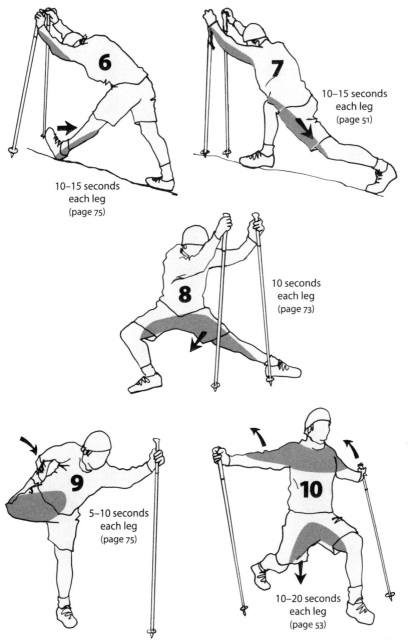

6

10–15 seconds
each leg
(page 75)

7

10–15 seconds
each leg
(page 51)

8

10 seconds
each leg
(page 73)

9

5–10 seconds
each leg
(page 75)

10

10–20 seconds
each leg
(page 53)

BEFORE & AFTER **TRIATHLON (SWIMMING)**

APPROXIMATELY 2 MINUTES

Walk for several minutes before stretching.

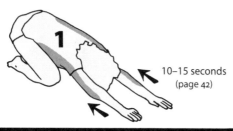

1 10–15 seconds
(page 42)

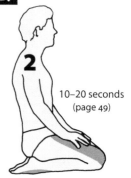

2 10–20 seconds
(page 49)

BEFORE & AFTER **TRIATHLON (CYCLING)**

APPROXIMATELY 1½ MINUTES

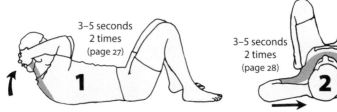

1 3–5 seconds
2 times
(page 27)

2 3–5 seconds
2 times
(page 28)

BEFORE & AFTER **TRIATHLON (RUNNING)**

APPROXIMATELY 2 MINUTES

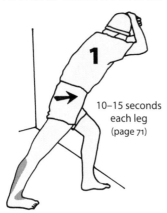

1 10–15 seconds
each leg
(page 71)

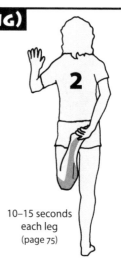

2 10–15 seconds
each leg
(page 75)

Stretching: Pocket Book Edition © 2021 by Bob and Jean Anderson. Shelter Publications, Inc.

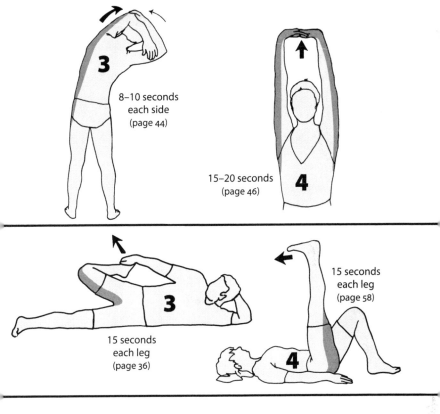

3 8–10 seconds
each side
(page 44)

4 15–20 seconds
(page 46)

3 15 seconds
each leg
(page 36)

4 15 seconds
each leg
(page 58)

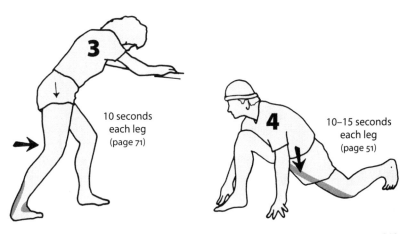

3 10 seconds
each leg
(page 71)

4 10–15 seconds
each leg
(page 51)

APPROXIMATELY 4 MINUTES

Walk or jog for 2–3 minutes before stretching.

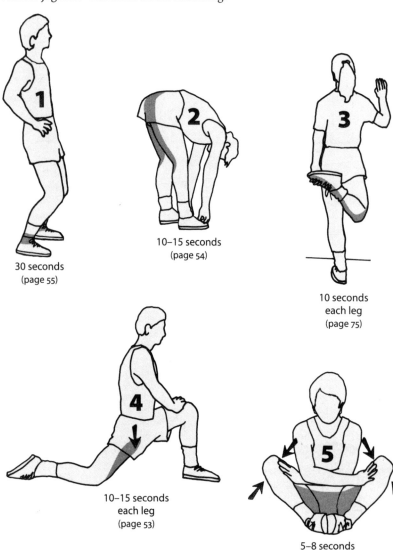

30 seconds
(page 55)

10–15 seconds
(page 54)

10 seconds
each leg
(page 75)

10–15 seconds
each leg
(page 53)

5–8 seconds
(page 59)

Stretching: Pocket Book Edition © 2021 by Bob and Jean Anderson. Shelter Publications, Inc.

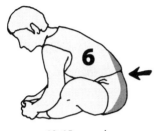

10–15 seconds
(page 58)

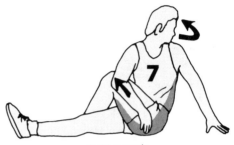

8–10 seconds
each side
(page 60)

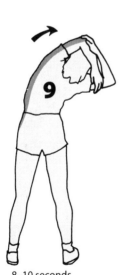

8–10 seconds
each side
(page 44)

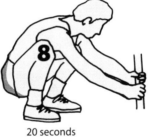

20 seconds
(page 66)

Mini-routine:
1, 4, 8, 9, 10
Approx. 2 min.

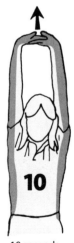

10 seconds
(page 46)

APPROXIMATELY 4 MINUTES

Warm up by using a stationary bike or treadmill, etc., for 3–5 minutes before stretching.

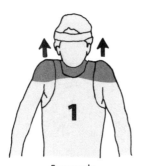

5 seconds
2 times
(page 46)

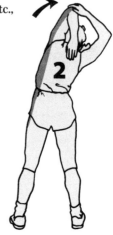

8–10 seconds
each side
(page 44)

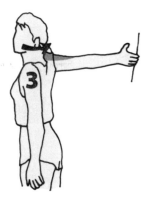

10 seconds
each arm
(page 82)

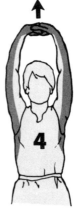

15 seconds
(page 46)

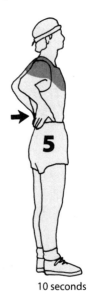

10 seconds
(page 46)

Stretching: Pocket Book Edition © 2021 by Bob and Jean Anderson. Shelter Publications, Inc.

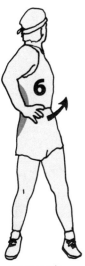

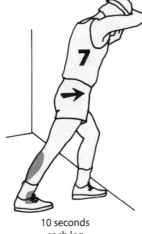

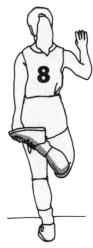

6

10 seconds
each side
(page 81)

7

10 seconds
each leg
(page 71)

8

10–15 seconds
each leg
(page 75)

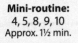

Mini-routine:
4, 5, 8, 9, 10
Approx. 1½ min.

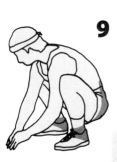

9

10–15 seconds
(page 66)

Stretch between
sets to promote
"active rest" and
to keep your
circulation moving.

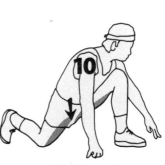

10

15–20 seconds
each leg
(page 51)

APPROXIMATELY 4 MINUTES

Walk for several minutes before stretching.

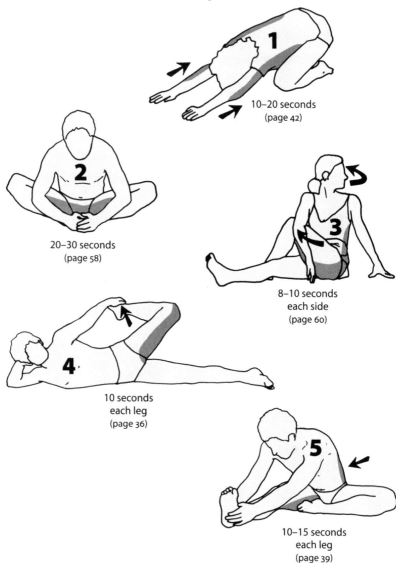

1 10–20 seconds
(page 42)

2 20–30 seconds
(page 58)

3 8–10 seconds
each side
(page 60)

4 10 seconds
each leg
(page 36)

5 10–15 seconds
each leg
(page 39)

Stretching: Pocket Book Edition © 2021 by Bob and Jean Anderson. Shelter Publications, Inc.

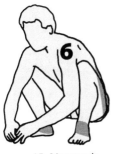

15–30 seconds
(page 65)

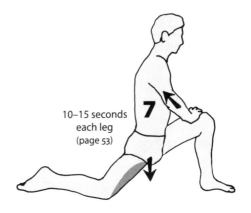

10–15 seconds
each leg
(page 53)

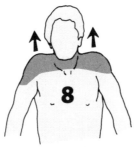

5 seconds
2 times
(page 46)

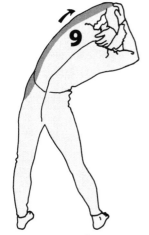

8–10 seconds
each side
(page 44)

Mini-routine:
8, 6, 7, 9, 10
Approx. 1½ min.

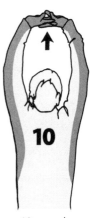

10 seconds
(page 46)

APPROXIMATELY 4 MINUTES

Jog for 2–3 minutes before stretching.

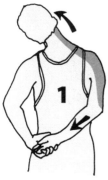

10 seconds
each arm
(page 47)

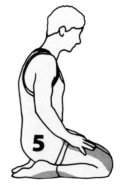

8–10 seconds
each side
(page 44)

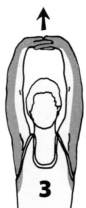

15 seconds
(page 46)

5 seconds
each arm
(page 42)

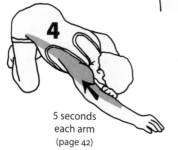

15–20 seconds
(page 49)

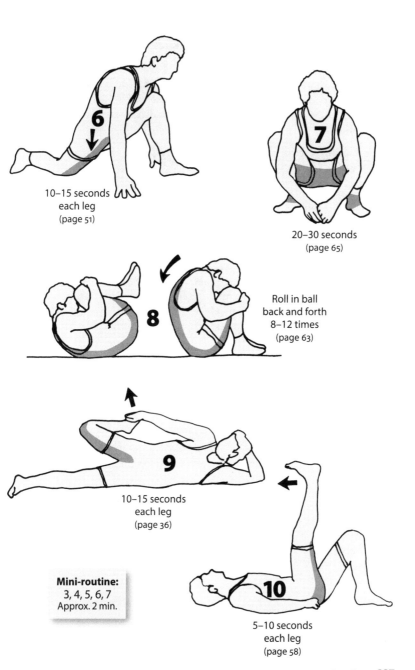

6

10–15 seconds
each leg
(page 51)

7

20–30 seconds
(page 65)

8

Roll in ball
back and forth
8–12 times
(page 63)

9

10–15 seconds
each leg
(page 36)

Mini-routine:
3, 4, 5, 6, 7
Approx. 2 min.

10

5–10 seconds
each leg
(page 58)

To Teachers and Coaches

For student athletes training has always stressed discipline, constantly pushing to new limits, and building maximum strength and power. As teachers and coaches, you are interested, of course, in team performance. But your most important goal is to educate the individuals under your supervision.

The best way to teach stretching is by your own example. When you yourself do the stretches and enjoy them, you will communicate this with enthusiasm. You will generate the same kind of attitude in your students.

In recent years, some attention has been given to stretching for injury prevention, but even here, there has been too much emphasis on maximum flexibility. *Stretching is entirely individual.* Let your students know that it is not a contest. There should be no comparisons made between students, because each is different. The emphasis should be on the feeling of the stretch, not on how far one can go. Stressing flexibility at the beginning will only lead to overstretching, a negative attitude, and possible injuries. If you notice someone who is tight or inflexible, don't single that person out; emphasize the proper stretches for that person alone, away from the group.

As a teacher/coach/guide, emphasize that stretching should be done with care and common sense. You do not have to set standards or push limits. Do not overwork or force your students to do too much. They will soon discover what feels right to them. They will improve naturally — and enjoy it.

It is important for students to understand that each and every one of them is an individual, with his or her own limits and a certain potential. All they can do is their best, nothing more.

The greatest gift you can give your students is to prepare them for the future. Teach them the value of regular exercise, of stretching daily, and of eating sensibly. Impress upon them that everyone can be fit, regardless of strength or athletic ability. Instill in your students an enthusiasm for movement and health that will last a lifetime.

APPENDIX

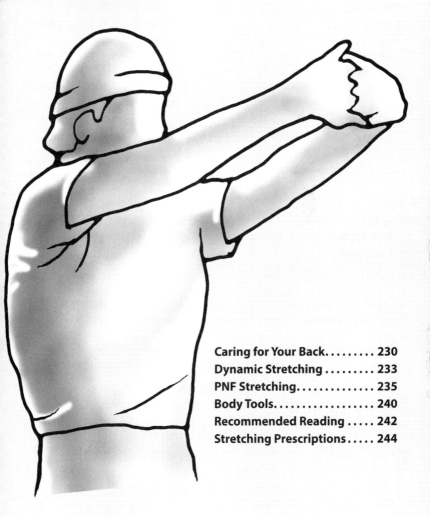

Caring for Your Back

More than 50 percent of all Americans will suffer from some sort of back problem some time during their lives. Some problems may be congenital, such as sway back or *scoliosis* (lateral curvature of the spine). Others may be the result of an automobile accident, a fall, or sports injury (in which case the pain may subside, only to reappear years later). But most back problems are simply due to tension and muscular tightness, which come from poor posture, being overweight, inactivity, and lack of abdominal strength.

Stretching and abdominal exercises can help your back if done with common sense. If you have a back problem, consult a reliable physician who will give you tests to see exactly where the problem lies. Ask your physician which of the stretches and exercises shown in this book would be of most help to you.

Anyone with a history of lower back problems should avoid stretches, called hyperextensions, that arch the back. They create too much stress on the lower back, and for this reason I have not included any such stretches in this book.

The best way to take care of your back is to use proper methods of stretching, strengthening, standing, sitting, and sleeping. For it is what we do moment to moment, day to day, that determines our total health. In the following pages are some suggestions for back care. *(Also see pp. 26–33.)*

Some Suggestions for Back Care and Posture

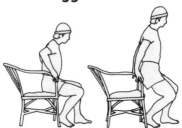 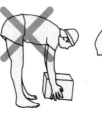 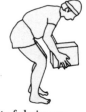

Never lift anything (heavy *or* light) with your legs straight. Always bend your knees when lifting something, so the bulk of the work is done by the big muscles of your legs, not the small muscles of your lower back. Keep the weight close to your body and your back as straight as possible.

Getting in and out of chairs can be a hazard to your back. Always have one foot in front of the other when rising from a chair. Move your bottom to the edge and, with your back vertical and chin in, use your thigh muscles and arms to push yourself straight up.

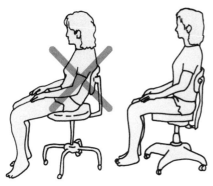

If your shoulders are rounded and your head tends to droop forward, bring yourself into new alignment. This position, when practiced regularly, will lessen back tension and keep the body fresh with energy. Pull your chin in slightly (not down, not up), with the back of your head being pulled straight up. Think of your shoulders being down.

Breathe with the idea that you want the middle of your back to expand outward. Tighten your abdominal muscles as you flatten your lower back into the chair. Do this while driving or sitting to take pressure off the lower back. Practice this often and you will naturally train your muscles to hold this more alive alignment without conscious effort.

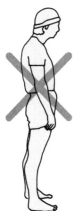

Do not stand with your knees locked. This tilts your hips forward and puts the pressure of standing directly on your lower back: a position of weakness. Let the quadriceps support the body in a position of strength. Your body will be more aligned through the hips and lower back with knees slightly bent.

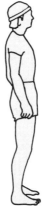

When standing, your knees should be slightly bent (½ inch), with feet pointed straight ahead. Keeping the knees slightly bent prevents the hips from rotating forward. Use the big muscles in the front of the upper legs *(quadriceps)* to control your posture when standing.

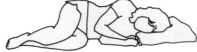

A good, firm sleeping surface helps in back care. If possible, sleep on one side or the other. Sleeping on your stomach can cause tightness in the lower back. If you sleep on your back, a pillow under your knees will keep your lower back flat and minimize tension.

If you stand in one place for a period of time, as when doing the dishes, prop one foot up on a box or short stool. This will relieve some of the back tension that comes from prolonged standing.

When you are aware that your posture is bad, automatically adjust into a more upright, energetic position. Good posture is developed through the constant awareness of how you sit, stand, walk, and sleep.

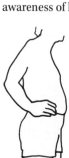

Many tight and so-called bad backs can be caused by excessive weight around the middle. Without the support of strong abdominal muscles, this extra weight will gradually cause a forward pelvic tilt, causing pain and tension in the lower back.

1. Develop the abdominal muscles by regularly doing abdominal curls. Exercise within your limits. It takes time and regularity. But if you don't get into it, the condition will only worsen.

2. Develop the muscles of the chest and arms by doing knee push-ups. These push-ups isolate the muscles in the upper body without straining the lower back. Start an easy three-set routine such as 10–8–6, or whatever — just get started!

3. Stretch the muscles in the front of each hip as shown on p. 51, and stretch the muscles of the lower back *(pp. 26–33 and 63–67)*. By strengthening the abdominal area and stretching the hip and back areas, you can gradually undo the forward pelvic tilt that is, in so many cases, the main cause of back problems.

4. Slowly let the size of your stomach shrink by not overeating.

5. Learn how to walk before you jog, and jog before you run. If you walk a mile a day (at one time) every day, without increasing your calorie intake, you will lose ten pounds of fat in one year.

A unique book on self-care for low-back pain:

Treat Your Own Back, by Robin McKenzie, published by OPTP <www.OPTP.com>, 2006.

Dynamic Stretching

What's all this you hear these days about "dynamic stretching?" There have been recent media articles claiming that "dynamic stretching" is the preferred method for athletes, that static stretching is no longer useful before competition, and in fact, may even be harmful. First, some definitions:

- *Dynamic* stretching is defined as "...actively moving a joint through the range of motion required for a sport."
- *Static* stretching refers to holding a stretch with no movement.
- Stretching, as in this book, refers to a two-phase stretch with movement.*

What's going on here? It may have started with a well-publicized study in the 1994 Honolulu Marathon in which runners who stretched had more injuries than those who didn't. First, how did the control group stretch? If incorrectly (as many competitors do — pushing too far, or bouncing), it could well have increased injuries. And why conclude that stretching *caused* the injuries? (Curiously, these results applied only to white males, not women or Asians.)

Some sports trainers say athletes should not practice static stretching *before* competition (although many of them recommend it *after* the event). Here's what I recommend:

For athletes: After a warm-up, some gentle stretches will prepare you for dynamic stretches, drills, and further warming up. Mild stretches give your muscle a signal they are about to be used. And, static stretching (two-phase) after the event is highly beneficial.

For the general population (ordinary people, not competitive athletes): I believe two-phase stretching is as effective and useful as ever. Over 3½ million people (worldwide) have bought and used *Stretching* (the great majority of them not competitive athletes). We've received favorable feedback for over 30 years. Stretching makes people *feel* better.

And what about yoga? Hundreds of millions of people throughout the world practice yoga, which is actually static stretching. Would they be practicing yoga if it wasn't beneficial?

———

*My type of stretching isn't strictly "static." It consists of a two-phase stretch: the *easy stretch,* where you relax into the stretch, is followed by the *developmental stretch,* where you move it a little farther — always paying close attention to how your body feels.

Curiously, if you check out dynamic stretches, many of them are really drills. Arm swings, leg swings, side bends, toe touches. Nothing new here; these movements have been used for years by athletes in warm-ups; they just weren't called "dynamic stretching."

Some of the new dynamic stretches look good to me, including those that take a regular stretch and add motion, mimicking sports-specific movements. You can see a video of these online at: *www.shltr.net/dynstretch*. If I were a competitive athlete, I'd look into dynamic stretching, and — listen to my coach or trainer. But I'd keep static stretches in my toolbox.

To say that dynamic stretching replaces static stretching is short-sighted. One doesn't replace the other, any more than Nautilus machines replaced free weights (or television replaced radio). They each have their place. The millions of people throughout the world who have used *Stretching* will continue to use and benefit from the book. Competitive athletes and their coaches will continue evolving warming-up and stretching techniques, finding the best combination for optimum performance and avoidance of injury.

Stretching for ordinary people (such as office workers or computer users) is about feeling your body, paying attention to stiffness and flexibility. Tune in to your body, never push things to the point of pain, never bounce, or do extreme stretches. Focus on how each stretch feels. Be sensitive to your body. You don't need a Ph.D. to tell you how you feel, any more than you "…need a weatherman to know which way the wind blows." Try some stretches *(for example, pp. 15–21)* and you be the judge.

PNF Stretching

PNF is the abbreviation for "proprioceptive neuromuscular facilitation," a physical therapy developed after World War II to help rehabilitate soldiers suffering from neurological disorders. By the '60s and '70s, physical therapists and sports trainers began using PNF techniques to increase flexibility and range of motion for healthy people, including athletes. In ensuing years, PNF practices have gained popularity with trainers and athletes seeking to optimize sports performance.

Though this book is primarily about two-phase, static stretching, I have also included some basic PNF stretches. PNF is most often used by athletes and by individuals who have less-than-normal range of motion or who have lost normal range of motion. The PNF stretches in this book can be done without a partner or assisting device. They are easy to learn and use. These stretches are mainly the *contract-relax-stretch technique* and the *antagonist contract-relax technique*. Following are descriptions and examples of these two types of PNF stretches.

Contract-Relax-Stretch Technique

Here the muscle is passively taken through a range of motion that produces a mild (not painful) stretch tension, then contracted (as forceful as a closed fist) for 4–5 seconds, then relaxed momentarily, and then taken once again into a mild static stretch for 5–15 seconds. This process may be repeated several times. Each time you can expect a slight increase in tension-free flexibility.

Isometric contraction — a muscular contraction in which you increase muscle tension, but the muscles do not lengthen and the joints do not move.

Important: Because of the moderate isometric contraction required in PNF, individuals with heart disease or high blood pressure should be cautioned in the use of PNF. (My approach to isometric contractions is to exert much less than maximal effort.)

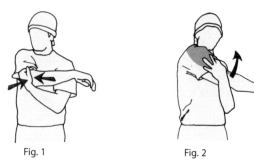

Fig. 1   Fig. 2

Pull your elbow across your chest until a mild (not painful) stretch is felt, then move your elbow away from your body against the resistance of your opposite hand. Now hold a sustained (50–60 percent) isometric contraction for 4–5 seconds *(fig. 1)*. (Do not hold your breath; breathe during contraction of the muscle you will be stretching next.) Relax momentarily and then use your hand and arm to pull your elbow further back across your chest until a mild stretch tension is again felt in the muscles just contracted *(fig. 2)*. Hold a mild (moderate) stretch for 5–15 seconds. Repeat several times.

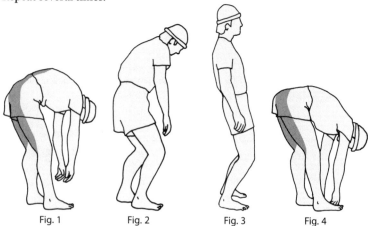

Fig. 1   Fig. 2   Fig. 3   Fig. 4

Antagonist Contract-Relax Technique

The second PNF technique uses the principle of contracting and relaxing opposing muscles, such as with the quadriceps (front thigh) and the hamstrings (back of thigh). In this PNF technique, you contract your quadriceps to relax your hamstrings, then stretch your hamstrings, as in figure 1 or 4. This action facilitates the hamstrings' relaxation through the reciprocal inhibition reflex. (Sounds complicated but is easy to do.) When you contract your quadriceps, as in figure 3, your hamstrings will relax.

Try it out. Start in a standing position and slowly bend forward from the hips (keeping knees slightly flexed), until you reach a comfortable stretch *(fig. 1)*. At this time note how far you are able to go. Return to a standing position, keeping your knees slightly flexed as you do so *(fig. 2)*.

Now assume a flexed-knee position, with feet flat and pointed straight ahead *(fig. 3)*. Hold for 15–20 seconds. This position contracts your quadriceps and relaxes your hamstrings, which should make it easier to stretch your hamstrings in the next position. Stand up straight and without bouncing go into the first stretch *(fig.1)*. Hold for 5–15 seconds or so. You will probably be able to stretch farther now than you could the first time with the same amount of effort. Repeat figures 3 and 1 several times and expect slight-to-moderate flexibility gains *(fig. 4)*.

These two examples should help you to understand and be able to use some basic PNF stretches. The PNF stretches are scattered throughout the book, being mixed in with the sustained (static) stretches. I think the combination of sustained (static) stretches and PNF stretches works quite well.

Caution: Do not overdo the PNF stretches. Stay relaxed and don't strain during mild contractions. Keep breathing! Be comfortable in your approach. Straining and overdoing only leads to not doing!

On the next two pages is a summary of PNF stretches that appear in various places throughout the book.

PNF STRETCHES

Here are some PNF stretches, as described in the preceding two pages. Try them out to see if the technique works for you (helps you get more flexible). Once you get the idea, you can use the technique on any stretch. Contract-relax-stretch, contract-relax-stretch, etc.

Repeat each of these series several times. Hold each contraction 4–5 seconds, each stretch 5–15 seconds.

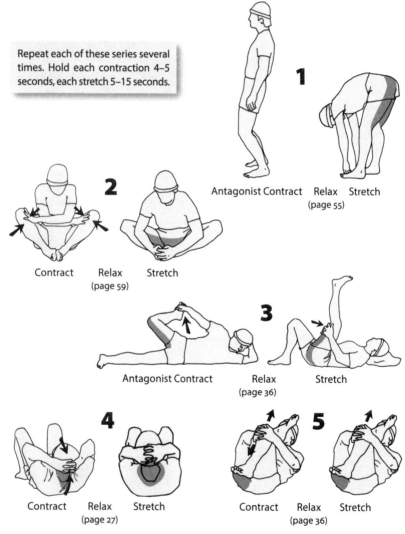

1

Antagonist Contract   Relax   Stretch
(page 55)

2

Contract   Relax   Stretch
(page 59)

3

Antagonist Contract   Relax   Stretch
(page 36)

4

Contract   Relax   Stretch
(page 27)

5

Contract   Relax   Stretch
(page 36)

   Stretching: Pocket Book Edition © 2021 by Bob and Jean Anderson. Shelter Publications, Inc.

Don't push it! No pain! *Feel* the stretch. Listen to your body.

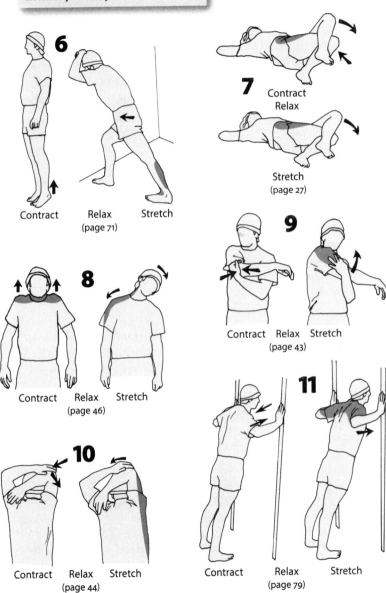

6

Contract   Relax (page 71)   Stretch

7 Contract Relax

Stretch (page 27)

8

Contract   Relax (page 46)   Stretch

9

Contract   Relax   Stretch (page 43)

10

Contract   Relax (page 44)   Stretch

11

Contract   Relax (page 79)   Stretch

Body Tools

Body tools are self-help devices that allow you to do body work (massage, acupressure) in a very precise way without a partner. I started using various body tools in the early '90s and found them really helpful. I also discovered that they worked exceptionally well when combined with regular stretching. So I introduced them to the participants at the camps I attended and clinics I gave and the response was excellent.

People like the fact that the tools are easy to use and that they are helpful with trigger points (knotted muscle tissue) and tension. They allow you to work on your body in completely different ways. You can easily access trigger points and sore spots. Tight muscle tissue can be loosened in just a few minutes with most of these tools. They make bodywork easy to do and pain reduction a reality.

Here are some tools that I use regularly and recommend.

TheraCane®

An acupressure tool that loosens tight, painful muscular areas. You use leverage and a slight downward pull to create the desired pressure wherever you want (mild pressure is recommended). Especially designed for the back of the neck, excellent for the mid-back (between shoulder blades), upper back, sides of neck, and shoulders. In fact, it can be used all over the body and even as a stretching aid. This tool has been extremely popular in many pain clinics throughout the United States. It's a great tool that many people find useful.

The Stick®

A non-motorized massage device used by serious athletes to loosen "barrier trigger points" (knotted-up muscles). The flexible core with revolving spindles easily molds to various body contours. This tool is wonderful for the legs, especially the calves, and can be used on all major muscle groups. You can use it through clothing or directly on the skin. The Stick provides instant myofascial release by relaxing healthy muscle fibers and promoting good circulation. Adequate blood supply allows muscles to feel better, work harder, last longer, and recover faster. Using this tool gets the muscles ready for activity, helps disperse lactic acid after a hard workout, helps prevent injuries, and hastens recovery time if injured.

The Breath Builder®

This device was originally designed for musicians to develop breath control; however it is excellent for anyone who wishes to develop restorative deep breathing. You blow into a tube and the pressure of your breath keeps a ping-pong ball afloat in the cylinder. It forces you to use your diaphragm muscles and to breathe correctly, with the goal of increasing your lung capacity. Taking more air into your lungs replenishes your bloodstream with oxygen and revitalizes every cell in your body (think of it!). The ball is a visual aid and tells you exactly what your diaphragm is doing by how high the ball floats in the cylinder. Comes with detailed instructions.

The Trigger Wheel®

A 2″ nylon wheel on a 4″ handle for deep massage. The Trigger Wheel works on trigger points (knotted muscles) and can be used directly on skin or through light clothing. It works the way a tire rolls back and forth on pavement. Very effective in reaching specific sore spots, such as small areas in the neck, hands, wrists, arms, legs, and feet. You can carry it with you and use it spontaneously throughout the day to keep pain at a minimum.

The Foot Massage®

A 2″ × 9″ roller with raised knobs for foot massage, and rubber rings to protect the floor. A super tool for tired feet. The studded knobs give you pinpoint access to the bottom of the foot. Used to stimulate nerve endings, reduce discomfort, and improve circulation. Use on the job if you sit a lot.

See p. 250 for information on ordering any of these tools.

Recommended Reading

8 Steps to a Pain-Free Back: Remember When It Didn't Hurt. Esther Gokhale, L.Ac.. Pando Press, Stanford, CA. 2008.

A revolutionary new book on improving posture and treating back pain. A wonderful approach.

The Alexander Technique: How to Use Your Body without Stress. Wilfred Barlow and Nikolaas Tinbergen. Inner Traditions, Int'l, Richester, Va. 1991.

An updated edition of the classic guide to F. M. Alexander's technique for successful body dynamics.

Awareness through Movement. Moshe Feldenkrais. Harper, San Francisco. 1991.

Illustrated, easy-to-use exercises to improve posture, vision, motivation, and self-awareness.

The Courage to Start: A Guide to Running for Your Life. John "The Penguin" Bingham. Simon & Schuster, New York. 1999.

An inspiring look at the struggles of a man in his 40s learning to run. Funny, witty, and compassionate. Great inspiration for anyone who wants to start running.

Galloway's Book on Running. Jeff Galloway. Shelter Publications, Bolinas, Calif. 2002.

This classic has helped many thousands of runners get started and train sensibly. It continues to be a best seller.

Getting Back in Shape. Bob Anderson, Ed Burke and Bill Pearl. Shelter Publications, Bolinas, Calif. 2007.

How to get back into shape. 30 programs, each with the three components of fitness: stretching, weight training, and moving exercises. A simple, visual approach to life-long fitness.

Getting Stronger: Weight Training for Sports. Bill Pearl. Shelter Publications, Bolinas, Calif. 2005.

Over half a million copies in print, this is 3 books in one: weight training for sports; bodybuilding; and general conditioning. The most complete book on weight training ever produced.

Healing Moves: How to Cure, Relieve and Prevent Common Ailments with Exercise. Carol Krucoff and Mitchell Krucoff, M.D. Healthy Learning, N.Y. 2009.

A timely book by an award-winning health columnist and a renowned cardiologist on the importance of vigorous exercise for general good health. Exercise relieves stress, keeps weight down, improves sleep and helps the body resist illness. There are exercise programs for general health and fitness, as well as exercise prescriptions for specific illnesses and health problems.

Myofascial Pain and Dysfunction, The Trigger Point Manual, Vol 1, Upper Half of Body; Vol 2, The Lower Extremities. Williams and Wilkins, Media, N.Y. 1999.

A classic. Beautifully illustrated. In-depth descriptions and solutions to myofascial pain and dysfunction through trigger point therapy. A reference book that is a pleasure to read and learn from.

Orthopaedic Sports Medicine: Principles and Practices. Jesse C. DeLee, M.D. and David Drez, Jr., M.D. W. B. Saunders Company, Philadelphia. 2009.

Experts in orthopaedic sports medicine share their experiences in dealing with sports injuries. The contributors give an excellent review of their topic, followed by their recommendations for treatment and recovery. These are not books for casual reading; the 2 volumes are over $350.

Running Within: A Guide to Mastering the Body-Mind-Spirit Connection for Ultimate Training and Racing. Jerry Lynch and Warren A. Scott. Human Kinetics, Champaign, Ill. 1999.

Dr. Lynch brings us to the forefront of sports psychology. Here are mental tools for running farther and faster, as well as for integrating body, mind, and spirit.

8 Weeks to Optimum Health. Andrew Weil, M.D. Ballntine Books, N.Y. 2007.

Dr. Weil believes in the body's natural abilities to heal. His changes are not radical but rather a series of simple, small steps to optimum health: taking supplements, adjusting eating habits, eliminating toxins from the diet, and an exercise program based on walking and improving breathing patterns.

Super Power Breathing: For Super Energy, High Health & Longevity. Paul C. Bragg and Patricia N. D. Bragg, Ph.D. Health Science, Goleta, Calif. 2008.

Excellent book on using your lungs to improve your health and increase your resistance to disease. A classic.

Touch for Health: A Practical Guide to Natural Health Using Acupressure Touch and Massage. John F. Thie. Devorss & Company, Marina del Rey, Calif. 2005.

How to utilize acupressure effectively, how to use kinesiology to test your body's need for foods, how to guide your own physical well-being. A complete system for home health.

Stretching in the Office. Bob Anderson and Jean Anderson. Shelter Publications, Bolinas, Calif. 2002.

Stretches and exercises for people who work in offices or at computers. Routines that will relieve stress and tension and keep the body tuned. Keep in your desk drawer.

STRETCHING PRESCRIPTIONS

Here is a summary of the stretches in this book that can be used by health care professionals when prescribing individual fitness and rehabilitation programs. Circle the stretches that are appropriate for the individual.

Relaxing Stretches for Your Back • 26–33

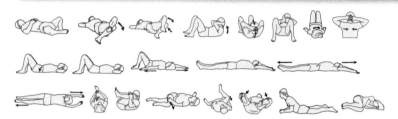

Stretches for the Legs, Feet, and Ankles • 34–41

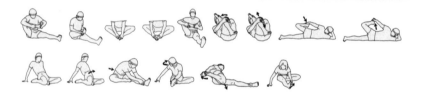

Stretches for the Back, Shoulders, and Arms • 42–48

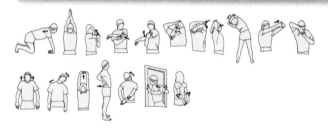

A Series of Stretches for the Legs • 49–53

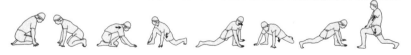

Stretches for the Lower Back, Hips, Groin, and Hamstrings • 54–61

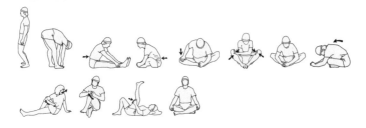

Stretches for the Back, Hips, and Legs • 63–67

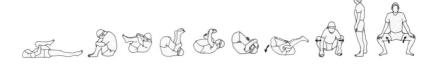

Elevating Your Feet • 68–70

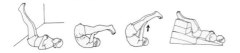

Standing Stretches for the Legs and Hips • 71–78

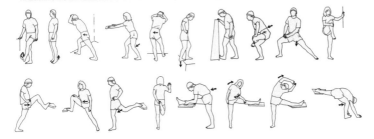

Standing Stretches for the Upper Body • 79–84

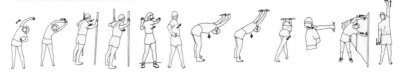

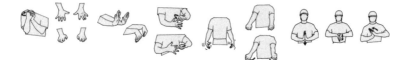
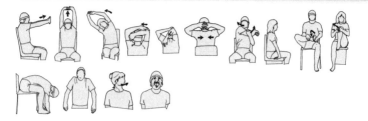
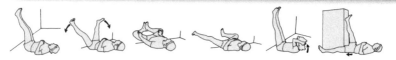
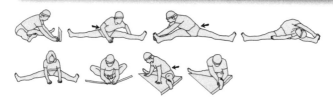
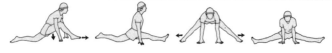

INDEX

247

MORE ON STRETCHING
FROM BOB AND JEAN ANDERSON

Over the past 35 years, Bob and Jean have developed a variety of their own stretching and fitness products, all designed to help people stay flexible and fit. In addition, Bob has discovered a number of body tools and workout products that are distributed by Stretching, Inc.

Stretching Charts

These large wall charts are great for learning how to stretch. They not only remind you to stretch (by being so visible), but guide you through a series of stretches (without having to look at the book). They come in both plain paper and laminated, and cover most of the routines in pp. 26–103 in this book.

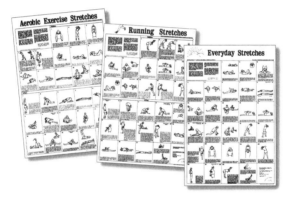

Stretching Chart Pads

These are miniature versions of the wall charts. They measure 8½ by 11 inches and come in pads of 40 identical sheets. As with the wall charts, full instructions are below each stretch. Used frequently by medical professionals, trainers, body workers, and coaches for their clients or team members.

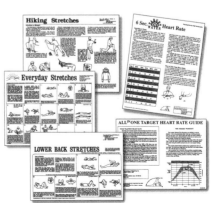

Stretching DVD

A 57-minute DVD organized in six comfortably paced sections: a brief introduction, stretches for the neck and back, then legs and hips, then feet, and finally, the arms and shoulders. The DVD and tape conclude with a 14-minute stretching routine for all body parts that can be used for everyday fitness or for sports. Suitable for people of all ages and interests. *(The DVD is in spoken English and Spanish; also available in VHS.)*

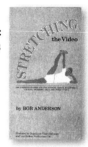

Stretch & Strengthen

This is a spiral-bound book for people in wheelchairs, the disabled, and the elderly. It contains stretching exercises and muscle-strengthening exercises performed with a circular resistive cord with tubular handles. Valuable for rehabilitation and for people with disabilities who want to increase their strength and flexibility.

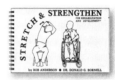

Body Tools

Body tools can be used in conjunction with stretching to help reduce muscular tension and pain. *(See pp. 240–241.)*

Shown here are:

TheraCane • The Foot Massage
Trigger Wheel • Breath Builder • The Stick

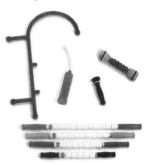

Maxit® Workout Gear

Functional sportswear for the person who wants warmth and dryness (97 percent wind-resistant) and breathability without layering. This blend of spun polyolefin (a new generation of polypropylene) and Lycra® is comfortable and durable. The clothing includes neckgators, balaclavas, sweatbands, headbands, undershirts, tights, shirts, socks. Great for all cold-climate activities.

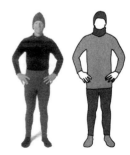

MORE WORLD-CLASS FITNESS BOOKS FROM SHELTER PUBLICATIONS

Two running books from Olympic runner Jeff Galloway, originator of the run walk run® method of training

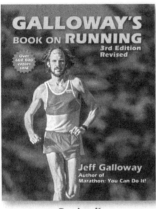

Revised!

Galloway's Book on Running
3rd Edition
Jeff Galloway

$21.95   7¼" × 9"
ISBN: 978-0-936070-85-8

- Now includes Jeff's run walk run® training method
- Over 600,000 copies sold

"Jeff Galloway is one of those rare individuals who not only knows his craft, but also has the ability to convey this knowledge through teaching."
—*Frank Shorter, Gold Medalist, 1972 Olympic Marathon*

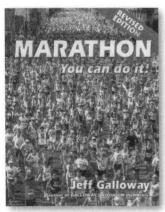

You can do it!

Marathon
You Can Do It!
Jeff Galloway

$18.95   7¼" × 9"
ISBN: 978-0-936070-25-4

- In the past 35 years, Jeff has coached tens of thousands of people to run their first marathon
- Over 100,000 copies sold

"If I can do it, anybody can. It really works!"
—*Rosemary Shannon (age 52)*

About the Authors

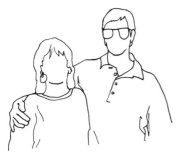

Bob Anderson is the world's most popular stretching authority. For over 35 years, Bob has taught millions of people his simple approach to stretching.

Bob and his wife Jean first published a home-made version of *Stretching* in a garage in southern California in 1975. The drawings were done by Jean, based on photos she took of Bob doing the stretches. This book was modified and published by Shelter Publications in 1980 for general bookstore distribution and is now known by lay people as well as medical professionals as the most user-friendly book on the subject. To date it has sold over 3¾ million copies worldwide and has been translated into 24 languages.

Bob is fit and healthy these days, but it wasn't always so. In 1968, he was overweight (190 pounds — at 5′9″) and out of shape. He began a personal fitness program that got him down to 135 pounds. Yet one day, while in a physical conditioning class in college, he found he couldn't reach much past his knees in a straight-legged sitting position. So Bob started stretching. He found he soon felt better and that stretching made his running and cycling easier.

The American fitness boom was just starting, and the millions of people who started working out were discovering the importance of flexibility in their fitness programs. After several years of exercising and stretching with Jean and a small group of friends, Bob gradually developed a method of stretching that could be taught to anyone. Soon he was teaching his technique to others.

He began with professional sports teams: the Denver Broncos, the Los Angeles Angels, the Los Angeles Dodgers, the Los Angeles Lakers, and the New York Jets. He also worked with college teams at Nebraska, UC Berkeley, Washington State, and Southern Methodist University, as well as other amateur and Olympic athletes in a variety of sports. He traveled around the country for years, teaching stretching to people at sports medicine clinics, athletic clubs, and running camps.

In the 1980s, Bob was a serious mountain runner and road biker. For ten years in a row he ran the Catalina Island Marathon in southern California, the 18-mile Imogene Pass run in Telluride, Colorado (which goes up over a 13,000-foot-high ridge), and the Pike's Peak Marathon. These days Bob spends most of his workout time on a mountain bike and hiking in the mountains above his house in Colorado, often going for 2–4 hour bike rides in the mountains, with occasional trips to Nevada. Though Bob works out a lot, he knows that training like this is not necessary for the average person to be fit. Through his travels, lectures, and workshops, he's kept in constant touch with people in all degrees of physical condition.

Jean Anderson has a B.A. in art from California State University at Long Beach. She began running and cycling (and stretching) with Bob in 1970. She developed a system of shooting photos of Bob doing the stretches, then making clear ink drawings of each stretch position. Jean was photographer, illustrator, typesetter, and editor of the first homemade edition of *Stretching*. These days she oversees Stretching Inc.'s mail-order business, and hikes and cycles to stay in shape.

CREDITS

Editor
Lloyd Kahn

Contributing Editor
Robert Lewandowski

Production Manager
Rick Gordon

Design
Rick Gordon
Jean Anderson

Cover Design
David Wills

Art Director
David Wills

Indexing
Frances Bowles

Proofreading
Robert Grenier

Models
Bob Anderson
Jean Anderson
Tiffany Anderson
Shari Boesel
Paul Comish
Kim Cooper
Debra Gentile
Karen Johnston
Bob Kahn
Will Kahn
Jim Melo
Justine Melo
Victoria Pollard
Christina Reski
Dave Roche
JoAnne Sercl
Kelsey Sercl
Shane Sercl
Mary Ann Shipstad
Shawntel Staab
Peggy Sterling
Joyce Werth

Printing
LSC Communications,
  Harrisonburg, Virginia, USA

Paper
Finch Opaque Vellum Book

Special thanks to the following
  people, who helped with this book
  in one way or another:
Joan Creed
Drake Jordan
Evan Kahn
Lesley Kahn
Mari Lillestol
Brian Roberts
Tess Rubinstein
Mary Sangster
George Young
The folks at Publishers Group West